Certified Hyperbaric Technologist Exam

CHT Test Review for the
Certified Hyperbaric Technologist Exam

Dear Future Exam Success Story:

Congratulations on your purchase of our study guide. Our goal in writing our study guide was to cover the content on the test, as well as provide insight into typical test taking mistakes and how to overcome them.

Standardized tests are a key component of being successful, which only increases the importance of doing well in the high-pressure high-stakes environment of test day. How well you do on this test will have a significant impact on your future, and we have the research and practical advice to help you execute on test day.

The product you're reading now is designed to exploit weaknesses in the test itself, and help you avoid the most common errors test takers frequently make.

How to use this study guide

We don't want to waste your time. Our study guide is fast-paced and fluff-free. We suggest going through it a number of times, as repetition is an important part of learning new information and concepts.

First, read through the study guide completely to get a feel for the content and organization. Read the general success strategies first, and then proceed to the content sections. Each tip has been carefully selected for its effectiveness.

Second, read through the study guide again, and take notes in the margins and highlight those sections where you may have a particular weakness.

Finally, bring the manual with you on test day and study it before the exam begins.

Your success is our success

We would be delighted to hear about your success. Send us an email and tell us your story. Thanks for your business and we wish you continued success.

Sincerely,

Mometrix Test Preparation Team

Need more help? Check out our flashcards at: http://MometrixFlashcards.com/Hyperbaric

Written and edited by the Mometrix Exam Secrets Test Prep Team
Printed in the United States of America

TABLE OF CONTENTS

Top 20 Test Taking Tips

1. Carefully follow all the test registration procedures
2. Know the test directions, duration, topics, question types, how many questions
3. Setup a flexible study schedule at least 3-4 weeks before test day
4. Study during the time of day you are most alert, relaxed, and stress free
5. Maximize your learning style; visual learner use visual study aids, auditory learner use auditory study aids
6. Focus on your weakest knowledge base
7. Find a study partner to review with and help clarify questions
8. Practice, practice, practice
9. Get a good night's sleep; don't try to cram the night before the test
10. Eat a well balanced meal
11. Know the exact physical location of the testing site; drive the route to the site prior to test day
12. Bring a set of ear plugs; the testing center could be noisy
13. Wear comfortable, loose fitting, layered clothing to the testing center; prepare for it to be either cold or hot during the test
14. Bring at least 2 current forms of ID to the testing center
15. Arrive to the test early; be prepared to wait and be patient
16. Eliminate the obviously wrong answer choices, then guess the first remaining choice
17. Pace yourself; don't rush, but keep working and move on if you get stuck
18. Maintain a positive attitude even if the test is going poorly
19. Keep your first answer unless you are positive it is wrong
20. Check your work, don't make a careless mistake

Minimum General Requirements

Effects of pressure exposure

Cardiovascular system

Hyperbaric oxygen therapy (HBOT) may affect the cardiovascular system. HBOT causes cardiac output to decrease by 24% to 35%. Pressure exposure inside the chamber will cause the blood vessels to vasoconstrict, decreasing blood flow to the body's tissues. This vasoconstriction results in a redistribution of blood flow (a hemodynamic change), so that the blood supply is not only maintained, but it also increases during hyperoxemia; including previously hypoxic areas. The pressure increase combined with the oxygen increase work together to improve oxygen tensions in the body tissues required for wound healing as well as other hyperbaric indication improvements.

Respiratory system

Pressure from a hyperbaric chamber may affect the lungs in a negative way. According to Boyle's law, as the pressure is increased, the volume is decreased, but as the pressure is decreased, the volume is increased. Therefore, if the patient holds his or her breath or stops breathing during the decompression phase of the chamber treatment, the lungs could burst from the sheer increase of volume. A burst lung, or a collapsed lung, is known as a pneumothorax. This is a life-threatening event that requires emergency procedures to be implemented by the hyperbaric staff.

Musculoskeletal system

Hyperbaric oxygen therapy may affect the musculoskeletal system. The musculoskeletal system has an increased sensitivity to ischemia, especially in a large muscle mass, and it can get necrotic very quickly after a trauma. Oxygen under pressure, such as in hyperbarics, affects the production and viability of free radicals, which can promote the healing of an ischemia/reperfusion (IR) injury. Microcirculation failure in skeletal muscle has been linked to IR injuries in a study of neutrophil adhesion to the capillaries. Microvascular perfusion is increased by hyperbaric oxygen therapy, thereby counteracting the ill effects of IR injuries. Vitamin E may prevent IR damage to the skeletal muscles.

Neurological system

Most neurological symptoms or deficits after a dive can be considered a manifestation of decompression sickness or arterial gas embolism and should be treated according to *U.S. Navy Diving Manual* treatment tables 5, 6, and 6A. Prevalent signs and symptoms are a feeling of detachment from reality and visual disturbances. In the event that these neurological manifestations persist after recompression, daily hyperbaric oxygen treatments may be required as long as improvement can be shown. The treatment indicated is 2.5 atmospheres absolute for 90 minutes while breathing 100% oxygen with air breaks. The patient may be treated once or twice a day for up to 14 days.

Formulas commonly used in diving and hyperbaric practice

Diving and hyperbaric operations use formulas to convert pressure measurements from feet of seawater (fsw) or meters of seawater (msw) to atmospheres absolute (ATA) or pounds per square inch gauge (psig) and pounds per square inch absolute (psia). Formulas are also used to convert temperature among Fahrenheit, Rankine, Celsius, and Kelvin.

Atmosphere absolute: $\text{ATA} = \frac{\text{fsw}}{33} + 1$

fsw to psi: $\text{psig} = \text{fsw} \times 0.445$ or $\text{psig} = \text{msw} \times 1.46$; $\text{psia} = \text{psig} + 14.7$

Temperature: $°\text{F} + 460 = °\text{R}$ and $°\text{C} + 273 = K$

Millimeters of mercury (mmHg) is another absolute pressure measurement often used in hyperbaric applications.

Millimeters of mercury: $\text{mmHg} = 760 \times \text{ATA} = 51.7 \times \text{psia}$

Calculating pressure, volume, or temperature

When using any of the below equations to calculate pressure, volume, or temperature, be sure to note that all pressures and temperatures used must be in absolute units (ATA, psia, or mmHg; and °R or K).

Boyle's law: $P_1V_1 = P_2V_2$ or $\frac{P_1}{V_2} = \frac{P_2}{V_1}$

Charles's law: $\frac{V_1}{T_1} = \frac{V_2}{T_2}$

Gay-Lussac's law: $\frac{P_1}{T_1} = \frac{P_2}{T_2}$

The general gas law: $\frac{P_1V_1}{T_1} = \frac{P_2V_2}{T_2}$

Various laws and their application to hyperbaric theory

Charles's law

Charles's law can apply to hyperbaric operations. Charles's law states that in a flexible container when the pressure remains constant, the temperature of a gas will be directly proportional to the volume of that gas. This means that when the temperature of a gas inside of a flexible container is increased, the volume will increase. Inversely, when the temperature is decreased, the volume will decrease as well. The formula for this law is $\frac{V_1}{T_1} = \frac{V_2}{T_2}$ or $V_1T_2 = V_2T_1$. This law applies only to flexible containers such as balloons or lungs in which the external pressure remains constant with volume changes. Remember to always convert your formula values to absolutes (Celsius to Kelvin or Fahrenheit to Rankine).

Graham's law

Graham's law states that different gases (in the body: carbon dioxide and oxygen) move from an area of high pressure to an area of low pressure independently of each other and at different rates to each other. This is the law of diffusion. Inside the lungs, oxygen is diffused through the alveolar membrane at a high concentration and oxygen is diffused through the blood at a low concentration, and at an even lower concentration in the tissues. Hyperbaric oxygen increases the diffusion rate and oxygen concentration in the entire body. In more technical terms, the rate of diffusion is inversely proportional to the square root of its molecular weight.

Pascal's law

Pascal's law states that if the pressure in a confined fluid is increased, the pressure at any point in that contained fluid will be equally increased. When applied to hyperbaric theory, Pascal's law means that a bubble deep inside the body's tissue will respond to the pressure outside the body. Pascal's law also applies to hydraulic systems in which incompressible fluids transmit force within the fluid from one area to another. The same principle applies to the human body when pressure is applied.

Various laws and their application to hyperbaric medicine practice

Boyle's law

Boyle's law can be defined this way: The pressure of a gas is inversely proportional to the volume of that gas, which means that if the pressure increased, the volume will decrease. In turn, if the pressure is decreased, the volume will increase. This is important to the hyperbaric technologist because the human body contains air spaces that can be affected by pressure changes, and pressure changes occur inside the hyperbaric chamber. You must inform the patient as a part of the education process to always breathe normally and to never hold their breath. The patient should also be shown multiple methods to clear the air space inside of the ears. When the pressure inside the hyperbaric chamber is increasing, the air spaces in the lungs and ears will grow smaller, and the ear air space will need to be relieved or cleared. If the patient is not breathing when the chamber pressure is decreased, the lungs will expand like a balloon and possibly burst. Therefore, it is important to monitor the patient closely and to communicate during all chamber pressure changes.

Dalton's law

Dalton's law, also known as the law of partial pressures, is defined as the sum of partial pressures in a mixture of gases equals the total pressure. This simply translates to the whole equals the sum of its parts. For example, the air we breathe is a mixture of nitrogen (78%), oxygen (21%), and other trace gases (1%). The pressure of this mixture is measured in units versus percentage, so in this case, 760 mmHg represents the total pressure at sea level. To calculate the pressure that each individual gas exerts, take the total pressure of the mixture and multiply it by the percent of that gas in the mixture. Oxygen's pressure would be 0.21 times 760, which equals 160 mmHg rounded. Nitrogen's pressure would be 0.78 times 760, which equals 593 mmHg rounded. Increasing the total pressure of a mixture of gases will also increase the pressure of each component gas.

Gay-Lussac's law

Gay-Lussac's law applies to the hyperbaric chamber operations. Gay-Lussac's law states that in a rigid container, when the volume remains constant, the pressure of a gas will be directly proportional to the temperature of that gas. This means that when the pressure of a rigid container is increased, the temperature will also be increased. Inversely, when the pressure of a rigid container is decreased, the temperature will be decreased. The formula for this law is $\frac{P_1}{T_1} = \frac{P_2}{T_2}$ or $P_1T_2 = P_2T_1$. The values in the formula must be converted to absolutes before calculating (Fahrenheit to Rankine, Celsius to Kelvin, psig to psia). This gas law only applies when the gas is inside a rigid container, such as a liquid oxygen converter or a scuba tank.

Henry's law

Henry's law can be applied to hyperbaric theory. Henry's law states that when the temperature is constant, the solubility of the gas inside of a liquid (bubbles) is directly proportional to the partial pressure of the gas directly above that liquid. To determine the solubility of a gas at a constant temperature, you must multiply the partial pressures of the gas by the Henry's law constant for the gas solution. This applies to hyperbaric theory when nitrogen bubbles dissolve in the blood during a deep dive. Decompression sickness may result if the nitrogen bubbles are not allowed to dissolve in solution from the blood properly. The solubility of a gas is determined by the equilibrium between the gas and the gas solution. The Henry's law constant is different for every gas.

Principles of heat transfer

Conduction

Heat conduction, also known as thermal conduction, happens through direct contact. When one object is in direct contact with another object and the first object is heated, heat energy is conducted from the first object to the second object. For example, a skillet is heated up on a stove. The attached handle of the skillet becomes very hot to the touch. The handle is heated through conduction. Some materials provide good conduction and are called conductors, while other materials provide poor conduction and are called insulators. Some materials that readily transmit or conduct energy (thermal conductors) are diamonds, silver, and gold. Some materials that insulate or do not readily conduct energy (thermal insulators) are water, plastic, wool, and foam. Electrical conductors include aluminum, silver, gold, and copper. Electrical insulators include air, plastic, rubber, and glass.

Convection

Heat convection is the transfer of heat energy through the currents of a fluid. The fluid is warmed through the collective movement of molecules in the fluid. The fluid becomes less dense allowing the movement of molecules to increase. For example, when water is heated in a pan, heat energy is transferred (convection) from the metal bottom of the pan into the water allowing the movement of the molecules. This movement of molecules starts at the bottom of the water in the pan and moves up, displacing the colder water molecules. Inside a monoplace hyperbaric chamber, a patient may become uncomfortably hot because of pressure change according to Charles's law, but the patient may also become hot because oxygen has a higher heat convection coefficient than air. The heat energy is transferred by convection through the skin into the outside environment. This is how a body cools itself. If the outside environment is warmer than the body's heat, other ways of cooling the body may be used.

Radiation

Heat radiation is a transfer of heat energy without a medium. This heat energy transfer is accomplished through electromagnetic waves or photons. The transfer of heat energy by radiation moves at the speed of light. The Sun heats up the Earth, but outer space is unaffected by heat from the Sun as the electromagnetic waves move through the vacuum of space. A car sitting in the heat of the Sun will be hotter than a car sitting inside of a garage, just as a decompression chamber without a roof to protect it from the Sun will be unbearably hot to the diver. Diver recompression in this example is not recommended. If a hyperbaric chamber inside of a facility is near to a window, the hyperbaric technologist's discretion is needed as to keeping the acrylic chamber out of direct sunlight. A patient who has confinement anxiety may request the window covering be opened. In this example, the technologist may use his or her discretion to decide whether to approve the patient's request depending on the time of day, weather, and temperature.

Importance of heat transfer to the hyperbaric technologist

The principle of heat transfer is important to know for the implementation of hyperbaric safety. Energy typically moves from a warmer system to a colder system. Heat is a form of energy. Specifically, heat is a form of kinetic energy and potential energy as it affects the seemingly random movement of molecules. The three principles of heat transfer are thermal conduction, thermal convection, and thermal radiation. As hyperbaric technologists, we use our understanding of heat to form and implement fire safety policies and to decide which materials and substances may be allowed inside of a hyperbaric chamber. There must be three elements present for a fire to occur: heat, fuel, and an oxidizer (the ignition), which is usually oxygen. Oxygen, although not flammable in and of itself, is a vital element for a fire to exist and thrive. The hyperbaric technologist cannot remove the oxygen because it is needed for patient treatment, but he or she can limit fuel and heat. Heat may come in the form of a tiny spark from an electronic device, i.e., a lighter that the patient forgot was inside a pocket or even an electrostatic shock. The predive safety checklist is in place for these very reasons.

Hyperbaric oxygen therapy process indicating air or gas embolism, decompression sickness

When a diver with decompression sickness is recompressed in a hyperbaric chamber, Boyle's law is applied. After exhibiting symptoms of decompression sickness and air or gas embolism, the diver is recompressed to a depth at which he feels relief. This is achieved through a pressure increase. An increase in pressure will decrease the volume of the bubbles of nitrogen inside the bloodstream, thus relieving the pain and pressure on the joints. The diver is treated on treatment tables 5, 6, and 6A of the *U.S. Navy Diving Manual* tables. Tables 5, 6, and 6A slowly and methodically bring the diver to the surface, thus giving the nitrogen bubbles a chance to diffuse into blood, exit through the lungs, and be exhaled from the body. The added benefit of breathing oxygen under pressure as opposed to air is that the amount of time needed to off-gas nitrogen is greatly reduced when breathing pure oxygen. The residual nitrogen in the body is diffused at different rates depending on the presence of fatty tissues and blood flow. This is why the knee might have pain, yet the elbow does not.

Hyperbaric oxygen therapy process

<u>Indicating carbon monoxide/cyanide poisoning</u>

Hyperbaric oxygen therapy should be implemented as early as possible when a patient presents with carbon monoxide (CO) poisoning or cyanide poisoning. Patients with a CO level of 25% in the hemoglobin are considered severely poisoned. Patients receive their first hyperbaric treatment at 3 atmospheres absolute (ATA) with 100% oxygen for about 2 hours, and are treated in the hyperbaric chamber at least two more times within the first 24-hour period. The half-life of CO in the hemoglobin while breathing air is 5.5 hours. When breathing 100% oxygen at 3 ATA, the half-life drops to 23 minutes. When the oxygen partial pressures are elevated, the CO becomes disassociated quickly from the hemoglobin.

Indicating clostridial myositis and myonecrosis

Gas gangrene is a necrotizing infection caused by bacteria that spreads rapidly when left untreated. This bacterium grows freely in oxygen tension of 30 mmHg and less, but growth is arrested or restricted at oxygen tensions of 70 mmHg and above. In animal studies, high concentrations of oxygen were found to arrest the effects of the necrotizing catalyst in gas gangrene. To effectively neutralize the deadly alpha toxins produced by the bacteria, hyperbaric treatment (three total dives) must be initiated within the first 24 hours of diagnosis. The first treatment is at 3 atmospheres absolute for 90 minutes while breathing 100% oxygen with air breaks. The next two treatments should be evenly spaced in the first 24-hour period.

Indications of crush injuries and skeletal muscle compartment syndrome

Crush injuries and skeletal muscle compartment syndrome are examples of acute traumatic ischemia. Hyperbaric oxygen therapy (HBOT) is an adjunctive treatment for traumatic ischemia. Oxygen tensions in the tissue become restricted in acute traumatic ischemia. HBOT restores and improves the tissue oxygen tensions, thereby initiating and improving wound healing. The hyperoxygenation of the red blood cells to capacity allows the plasma to onload oxygen and therefore oxygenate otherwise ischemic tissues. A secondary effect of HBOT is the vasoconstriction of the blood vessels, which has the effect of significantly reducing the edema produced from the traumatic ischemic injury.

Indication of infectious diseases

Hyperbaric oxygen (HBO) is very effective in the treatment of infectious diseases. HBO therapy works by inhibiting microbial growth and killing bacteria through increased oxygen tensions. HBO by itself is an effective antibacterial agent, but only at pressures above 1.5 atmospheres absolute. HBO is responsible for indirectly influencing infection outcomes by healing and repairing necrotic tissues. Room-air oxygen tends to enhance the growth of some aerobic bacteria, but HBO will inhibit that same bacteria. HBO increases the generation of free radicals, which are lethal for certain microorganisms, and they block the transport of ribonucleic acid substrates, therefore inhibiting the protein synthesis of bacteria.

Indication of severe anemia

Exceptional blood loss anemia is the loss of red blood cells, or hemoglobin, to the effect that the circulating of the blood can no longer meet the oxygen demand of the tissues. Hyperbaric oxygen therapy can meet the oxygen demands of the tissues when there is not an efficient means of a patient blood transfusion, or when there is a religious objection to blood transfusion. When the hemoglobin is 100% saturated with oxygen, the plasma can then onload oxygen in hyperbaric conditions. At 2 atmospheres absolute, the plasma can deliver up to 16.4 liters of oxygen at only a 60-minute treatment. This number goes up significantly when the treatment time is extended.

Indicating intracranial abscess

An intracranial brain abscess is an area in the brain where pus has accumulated. Typical criteria for use of hyperbaric oxygen therapy (HBOT) on an intracranial abscess are anaerobic or mixed pathogens, multiple abscesses, an abscess in a deep or dominant location, a compromised host, contraindicated surgery, and no surgical response. If the infection is life threatening, HBOT treatments are initiated early, and typically started at 2.5 to 3 atmospheres absolute, twice daily. HBOT is used as an adjunctive treatment, secondary to neurological surgery. Intracranial abscesses are typically composed of mainly anaerobic bacteria. Hyperbaric oxygen is an effective antibacterial agent.

Indicating necrotizing soft tissue infections

Necrotizing soft tissue infections are typically caused by aerobic, anaerobic, and mixed bacterial floras. These issues are increase in immunocompromised patients. Hyperbaric oxygen (HBO) is an adjunctive therapy secondary to surgical debridement, along with a course of antibiotics and good nutritional support. The tissues affected by a necrotizing infection must be oxygenated in order to kill the toxins and free the wound of bacteria. The goals of supersaturating the blood through HBO are improving wound healing through increased partial pressures of oxygen in the tissues, using higher oxygen tensions as a bacteria-killing agent, diminishing edema, and increasing circulation.

Indicating osteomyelitis (refractory)

Chronic refractory osteomyelitis (CROM) is a bone infection that cannot heal on its own. The three indications of CROM are a compromised host, a nonhealing fracture, and it is the diffuse sclerosing type. Osteomyelitis becomes chronic and refractory after treatment has occurred and it either persists or recurs. Oxygen tension in the bone is typically 25 mmHg. Under hyperbaric oxygen conditions, the oxygen tension is raised from 30 to 1200 mmHg, even in infected tissue. The raised oxygen tension increases the oxygen-dependent intracellular killing mechanisms, and reduces the number of organisms. Hyperbaric oxygen is used as an adjunctive therapy secondary to antibiotics and debridement.

Indicating delayed radiation injury

Radiation treatments are concentrated in a certain area to kill and reduce tumors, but even so, injury to normal tissues often occurs. Radiation injuries do not allow the normal revascularization that occurs in normal injuries. Radionecrosis may occur if the radiation is high enough. Hyperbaric oxygen therapy (HBO) helps to create capillary angiogenesis and fibroplasia. The mechanism of HBOT on radiated tissue is accomplished through wound healing and revascularization. A therapeutic dose of hyperbaric oxygen for soft-tissue radiation injuries is typically 2.5 atmospheres absolute for 90 minutes with two 5-minute air breaks. These treatments are given consecutively five days a week for 20 to 40 treatments. Transcutaneous oxygen measurements are used to track the progress and efficacy of the HBO treatments. HBO therapy is an adjunctive treatment secondary to surgery. Surgery may take place after 20 hyperbaric treatments.

Indicating compromised grafts and flaps

Skin grafts and flaps often become compromised when an arteriovenous shunt develops distally from the graft or flap. This shunt limits or shuts off blood flow, creating an area of hypoxia. The capillaries in the hypoxic area start to die off from lack of oxygen, and thus failure of the skin graft or flap occurs. Hyperbaric oxygen therapy (HBOT) causes vasoconstriction and greater blood flow. The increased flow of hyperoxygenated blood to the hypoxic area creates new capillaries and helps to close off the shunt that was limiting the flow of blood. HBOT has the ability to help collagen synthesis and fibroblasts that contribute to skin graft and flap survival. HBOT treatments for compromised skin grafts and flaps are typically given at 2 ATA for 90 minutes with no air breaks. Treatments are scheduled at five days a week for around 20 sessions.

Indicating a diabetic foot ulcer

Diabetes mellitus typically complicates wound healing through two mechanisms: (1) atherosclerosis and (2) defective cellular and humoral immunity. The effects of these mechanisms are chronic pedal ischemia, which results in lowered ability to fight infection and wound healing impairment, and decreased immunity leading to an increase in inflammatory processes. A diabetic foot ulcer may develop through a variety of factors. Diabetic neuropathy, which causes diminished pain in the feet, can lead to deformation of the foot by the denervation of the motor nerves. The absence of pain and the deformation of the foot can lead to wounding and subsequent infection. Transcutaneous oximetry is used to assess the oxygenation and perfusion of the tissue locally. Transcutaneous oxygen measurements are an evaluation tool to assess the healing potential of hyperbaric oxygen therapy (HBOT). HBOT will significantly increase the oxygen tension of the tissue, thus increasing collagen synthesis and fibroblast replication for optimal healing potential.

Barotrauma and all of the spaces in the body where it may occur

Any damage to the body tissues caused by a change in pressure is referred to as barotrauma. Barotrauma may occur in the hyperbaric chamber upon descent or ascent. The spaces in the body where air or gas may become trapped are susceptible to barotrauma with a change in pressure. According to Boyle's law, gases will increase in volume upon ascent, and gases will decrease in volume upon descent. The hyperbaric technologist should be aware where these pressure changes occur inside the body. A barotrauma will occur inside an enclosed gas-filled space, surrounded with a membrane lining, and consisting of an arterial blood supply that may be forced into the space to compensate for the ambient pressure change. The most common type of barotrauma is the middle ear squeeze. Other barotraumas are comprised of squeezes: the sinus squeeze, a tooth squeeze, an external ear squeeze, a lung squeeze, a body or face squeeze (from scuba gear), and an inner ear squeeze. If the gas from these enclosed spaces is not vented properly, tissue damage will result.

Effects caused by changes in pressure

A change in pressure on the human body may result in barotrauma. Any body cavity where a space of gas resides will be affected by pressure. According to Boyle's law, when pressure is increased, the volume of air or gas inside a body cavity will decrease. This causes a body cavity such as the middle-ear space, for example, to become smaller. Likewise, when the pressure is decreased, the volume of air or gas will increase, causing a body cavity space to grow larger. Barotrauma, trauma to the body tissues from the effects of pressure changes, may take place in descent or ascent, but it occurs mostly in descent. A squeeze is when barotrauma occurs on descent, and a reverse squeeze is when barotrauma occurs on ascent. When descending, a patient must equalize the pressure in the middle-ear space; when ascending, the middle-ear space is usually vented out through the eustachian tube on its own. The pressure will increase, however, if the tube is blocked. This pressure will attempt to relieve itself by bowing the eardrum outward, causing pain. A squeeze or a reverse squeeze may occur in any part of the body where air or gas may become trapped.

Use of a myringotomy

If a patient inside the hyperbaric chamber cannot equalize the pressure in the middle ear (ear squeeze), the patient may require pressure equalization tubes to be inserted by a physician. If the barotrauma in the middle ear is further complicated by acute otalgia (earache or ear pain), the patient may require a myringotomy. A myringotomy is a surgical procedure in which a small incision is made in the tympanic membrane so that gas may flow freely in and out of the eardrum. An unconscious patient being pressurized does not require a myringotomy.

Type 1 decompression illness (DCI), and associated signs, symptoms and risks

Decompression Illness (DCI) occurs when nitrogen is not given enough time to off-gas as a diver ascends from pressure. The nitrogen forms bubbles that may get lodged anywhere in the body if not dissolved properly. DCI may occur on any dive and at any time during the diver's career. There are two types of DCI: type 1 (pain only) and type 2 (serious symptoms). Type 1 symptoms include the following: rash (mark it with the time to track), itching (skin bends), pain in the extremities, lymph-node swelling (72 sets of lymph nodes in the body), marbling (discoloration of skin). Type 1 DCI is treated with treatment table 5: dive to 60 feet of seawater (fsw) at 20 feet per minute (fpm) for 10 minutes, and then dive to 30 fsw for two periods. If there is not 100% relief in 10 minutes, the treatment becomes a table 6 scenario: Dive to 60 fsw at 20 fpm for two periods, and then dive to 30 fsw for two periods.

Type 2 decompression illness, and associated signs, symptoms, and risks

Decompression illness (DCI) occurs when nitrogen is not given enough time to off-gas as a diver ascends from pressure. The nitrogen forms bubbles that may get lodged anywhere in the body if they are not dissolved properly. DCI may occur on any dive and at any time during the diver's career. There are two types of decompression illness: type 1 (pain only) and type 2 (serious symptoms). Type 2 symptoms include the following: fatigue; weakness; numbness; paresthesia (a tingling, creeping sensation on the skin); decreased sensation to touch; muscle weakness; paralysis; mental status changes; motor performance alterations; personality changes; bizarre behavior; lightheadedness; lack of coordination; tremors; disruption of urinary function; tinnitus (ringing in the ears); hearing loss; vertigo; dizziness; nausea; and vomiting. To treat type 2 DCI, treatment table 6 is used: Dive to 60 fsw at 20 fpm for two periods, and then dive to 30 fsw for two periods. However, if there is no relief after 20 minutes, the treatment becomes a table 6A scenario, which is a depth of 165 fsw at a rate of 20 fpm with two periods at 60 fsw and two periods at 30 fsw while looking for a point of relief.

Aspects of diving and hyperbaric medicine

Blood cells

Hyperbaric oxygen has an effect on the blood cells. During a treatment in the hyperbaric oxygen chamber, the body's red blood cells are supersaturated with oxygen allowing the blood plasma to onload oxygen as well. Hyperbaric oxygen also increases the deformability of the red blood cells, allowing them to flow through semiblocked blood vessels. The rate of perfusion is highly increased when the supersaturated red blood cells and the blood plasma flow to the capillaries. Even though the blood vessels are vasoconstricted by the hyperbaric pressure, the hyperbaric oxygen is still able to positively affect the perfusion rate.

Neurological system
There is an interest in treating neurological disease such as cerebral ischemia, or stroke, with hyperbaric oxygen therapy. Neural tissue is extremely sensitive to hypoxia, so it follows that hyperoxygenation of the brain would be beneficial. If the neural tissue does not receive an adequate vascular supply due to an occlusion of the cerebral blood vessels, an ischemic stroke may occur. Neurons can die in a matter of minutes when the blood supply is cut off. The cells of the penumbra part of the brain may be saved if adequate perfusion is restored because they remain viable for a prolonged period of time. Hyperbaric oxygen is known to improve perfusion, but this indication is still under consideration and is not yet approved by the Food and Drug Administration for hyperbaric oxygen therapy.

Cardiovascular system
Patients with suspected or established heart disease must undergo testing prior to initiating hyperbaric oxygen therapy, even though cardiac arrest inside the chamber is rare. These tests must at least include an electrocardiogram and if the patient has congestive heart failure, an echocardiogram must be performed. If the echocardiogram reveals an ejection fraction of less than 30%, the patient is contraindicated for hyperbaric oxygen therapy. If the patient has a cardiac arrest inside the monoplace chamber, have a code team standing by, and bring the patient out immediately upon a hyperbaric physician's order. A patient with a cardiac arrest inside a multiplace chamber has the added benefit of cardiopulmonary resuscitation being administered by the inside tender prior to depressurization.

Respiratory system
The presence of carbon dioxide in the body's tissues prompts the inhalation of gases, thereby completing the oxygen/carbon dioxide exchange. There is risk if a patient with chronic obstructive pulmonary disease, or other lung disease is placed in an atmosphere containing 100% oxygen. Insensitivity to carbon dioxide may not prompt the patient to breathe, leading to the loss of their respiratory drive. These patients should be watched closely during their hyperbaric oxygen treatments, especially the first treatment to be sure they are breathing adequately. The hyperbaric technologist may need to remind the patient to inhale or to take deeper breaths.

Ear squeeze and other barotraumas

Ear squeezes (barotrauma to the middle ear) are very common inside the hyperbaric chamber. Risk factors include anxiety, congestion, language barrier issues, irritants such as smoking, prior radiation treatment, and unconsciousness, to name just a few. Patients who have difficulty clearing their ears in the chamber may elect to have pressure equalizer (PE) tubes placed in the tympanic membrane. During the first hyperbaric treatment, a patient may have trouble clearing their ears. Hyperbaric technologist assistance in the prevention of middle-ear barotrauma starts before the patient enters the chamber. The technologist should reiterate equalization maneuvers right before the dive. The patient should know to equalize early and often. If the patient cannot clear during the treatment, the technologist may stop travel and lower the pressure by 2 psi, wait until the pain subsides, and try to pressurize again. This procedure may be repeated three times before aborting the treatment altogether. If the treatment is aborted because of barotrauma, the physician and the patient may opt for PE tubes or decongestants.

Carbon dioxide retention

The amount of carbon dioxide that a patient may rebreathe inside a multiplace hyperbaric chamber should be limited by the use of an oxygen hood or mask. If the hood or mask is malfunctioning or if the patient is not receiving 100% oxygen, carbon dioxide retention may occur and lead to an oxygen-toxicity seizure. The effect of carbon dioxide retention is usually not an issue in the hyperbaric chamber because the red blood cells are too supersaturated with oxygen to carry any carbon dioxide. Carbon dioxide is 50 times more soluble than the oxygen, so it dissolves in solution and is carried in the blood plasma. The plasma also carries oxygen inhaled from the pure oxygen atmosphere.

Carbon monoxide poisoning

Carbon monoxide (CO) poisoning may be treated with hyperbaric oxygen therapy at a pressure of 3 atmospheres absolute (ATA) for 90 minutes with air breaks, followed by two treatments of 2 ATA for 90 minutes in the first 24 hours. Treatments should be given 4 hours apart. Special attention must be paid to the risk factor of oxygen toxicity. Be ready to switch the patient to air at the first sign of oxygen toxicity. The symptoms to watch for are as follows: vision changes, ear ringing, nausea, tingling/twitching, irritability, dizziness, and convulsions (acronymized as VENTID-C). In the event of a seizure, stop the chamber travel and notify the hyperbaric physician and nurse. Watch for the patient's chest movement to observe normal or even irregular breathing. This indicates that the patient has passed the tonic phase of the seizure and entered the jerking, clonic phase, at which point you may bring the patient to the surface.

Hyperbaric chamber atmosphere and built-in breathing system contamination

Atmospheric contamination inside the monoplace hyperbaric chamber and the built-in breathing system is rare and may occur if the air tanks are contaminated and/or the liquid oxygen is not tested for purity at regular intervals. Atmospheric contamination inside the multiplace hyperbaric chamber may occur if the intake for the air compressor is not placed appropriately and not tested or maintained at regular intervals. If the patient breathes contaminated gas inside the chamber, the effects may be negative. For example, breathing carbon dioxide in excess may make the patient more susceptible to oxygen-toxicity seizures. Pressure tends to increase the effects of most gases.

Oxygen (O_2) toxicity

Hyperbaric technicians should be familiar with the signs and symptoms of oxygen toxicity in order to be able to recognize and respond to an occurrence. The prevention of oxygen toxicity includes knowing when a patient might be more susceptible to it, such as during a high fever or when taking certain medications. Most relative contraindications concerning oxygen toxicity may be resolved by medication or air breaks in the hyperbaric chamber. If the patient has oxygen toxicity and experiences a seizure inside the chamber, do not attempt to bring the patient to the surface because the patient will not be breathing during the seizure (it usually lasts about two minutes). If the signs and symptoms are noticed by the technologist or the patient before a seizure occurs, switch the patient's breathing gas to air immediately in an attempt to prevent the seizure.

Pressure-related issues

Anoxic and hypoxic events

Hypoxia (less than normal oxygenation) and anoxia (no oxygenation) have a negative effect on wound healing. If a wound is not curing, it is typically not receiving any oxygen, or it is not receiving enough oxygen to promote wound healing. The blood vessels carry the red blood cells full of oxygen to the tissues throughout the body. If oxygen is not reaching the wound, then neither is the blood; so that usually means a blood vessel must be blocked or occluded. Hyperbaric oxygen therapy works to supersaturate the red blood cells causing oxygen to be carried by the plasma as well, allowing the wound to be oxygenated once again.

Nitrogen

Nitrogen (N_2) is an inert gas that makes up the bulk (71%) of air. When making a dive on air to greater than 33 feet, a diver becomes susceptible to decompression sickness. At 33 fsw, the N_2 bubbles grow larger and take longer to dissolve in solution, causing pain and other symptoms of decompression sickness. The other effect of N_2 occurs when diving deeper than 100 fsw, and it is called N_2 narcosis. N_2 and other heavy, inert gases are soluble in lipid and exert an anesthetic effect. This is an effect of pressure that causes edema in the neuron cell membrane, disrupting the protein channels that regulate sodium and potassium. In this way, the neuron cell becomes permeable to ion transport. The N_2 effect limited divers to a depth of 300 fsw until further discoveries were made concerning lighter gas diving.

Vision changes

Changes in vision may occur in a patient undergoing a prolonged hyperbaric oxygen therapy treatment course. The pressure changes are presumed to change the shape of the lens, or they cause a change in refraction. These vision changes may cause symptoms such as blurry vision when staring at distant objects or a greater ability to focus on near objects. These causes are a result of myopia (near sightedness) as a side effect of hyperbaric oxygen therapy. The vision change usually only occurs in patients diving to 2.5 atmospheres absolute or greater. The myopia typically resolves from six weeks to three months after the last hyperbaric treatment.

Hypothermia versus hyperthermia

A human body going under pressure will experience temperature changes due to the changes in volume and pressure. This is in accordance with Gay-Lussac's law of pressure and temperature and Charles's law of volume and temperature. A diver who is making decompression stops inside a recompression chamber may experience hypothermia or hyperthermia, usually depending on the weather. If the water and weather are cold, the diver may experience hypothermia inside the chamber. The diver will already be stripped of the dive suit before entering the chamber. The diver should be sent in the chamber with towels and blankets to keep warm. One benefit of hypothermia under pressure is a possible deterrent to oxygen toxicity if the body has passed the point of shivering. A recompression chamber under the hot Sun could provide for hyperthermia in a recompressed diver. The diver should be given enough water to last throughout the chamber decompression time.

Gas Systems

Standard procedures for the use of gas

Chamber operations
Monoplace and multiplace hyperbaric chambers incorporate a gas breathing system. This gas breathing system must be monitored for safety. Liquid oxygen, air tanks, gas lines, fittings, valves, regulators, hoods, and masks are all part of the gas breathing system. These components must be inspected regularly. All gas valves should be opened and closed slowly. The oxygen supply is pressure controlled and flow regulated. High pressure (2000 to 3000 psi) is reduced through the regulator. Low pressure (approximately 200 psi) is controlled by the flowmeter. The flowmeter controls the amount of gas delivered to the patient's hood or mask. The hoods and masks must have tight seals and an overboard dump to vent out the exhaled carbon dioxide.

Life support systems
The monoplace hyperbaric chamber is filled and pressurized with 100% oxygen, whereas the multiplace chamber is pressurized with air. The monoplace chamber is constantly vented to prevent carbon dioxide contamination. The multiplace chamber has gas analyzers to determine the quality and content of the gases inside the chamber. Each chamber occupant inside the multiplace chamber contaminates the chamber atmosphere by exhaling approximately 3 cfm (cubic feet per minute) of carbon dioxide. A carbon dioxide scrubber must be installed to "wash" the air during treatment. The multiplace chamber must also be vented to keep the amount of oxygen below 23.5% for fire safety reasons. The gas analyzers must be constantly monitored by the chamber operator.

Chamber classifications

There are three types of hyperbaric chambers. Class A, or multiplace, hyperbaric chambers are used for human occupancy and may treat multiple patients at the same time. Class B, or monoplace, hyperbaric chambers are used for human occupancy and may only treat one patient at a time. Finally, a class C chamber is a non-human-occupancy chamber, usually for horses and other animals. A human must not be treated in a class C chamber; neither must an animal be treated in a class A or class B chamber.

Testing procedure for the purity and oxygen content of gases

To test for purity and oxygen content of gases inside the multiplace hyperbaric chamber, a gas analyzer must be used. Gas analyzers detect the concentrations of oxygen, carbon dioxide, and carbon monoxide. Gas analyzers are generally calibrated in the same fashion. An electrical current generates when the sensor is exposed to oxygen. This sensor must be exposed to the ambient air and the display must be adjusted to 20.9%. Daily calibration is required for most gas analyzers. Some analyzers require a special gas mixture for calibration. For example, a zero gas (nitrogen) and a full-scale gas (100% oxygen) may be used to calibrate an analyzer that uses a special mix in the midrange of the analyzer scale. The gas inside a multiplace chamber may be analyzed multiple times throughout the treatment.

Mathematical terms of gas usage

Breathing gas systems for hyperbaric operations are pressure controlled and flow regulated. The high pressure (2000 to 3000 psi) is reduced by a regulator to a working low pressure (200 psi) to feed a flowmeter for patient use. The inside tender for a multiplace chamber may use a demand mask to breathe, which requires 60 to 100 psig, and it consumes approximately 0.3 actual cubic feet per minute (acfm). The multiplace patient may use a hood to breathe in, which consumes 1.2 to 1.5 acfm, and it requires an overboard dump and a tight seal to prevent a high oxygen concentration inside the chamber atmosphere. Gay-Lussac's law is the law of pressure and temperature. The formula is $P_1/T_1 = P_2/T_2$, or $P_1T_2 = P_2T_1$. Be sure to use absolutes when calculating conversions. As the temperature rises, the pressure rises as well. When the liquid oxygen is converted to a gas in a rigid container, the temperature rises, and so the pressure rises. This conversion needs to be cooled.

Use of gas analyzers in a multiplace chamber

A gas analyzer is used by the hyperbaric technologist to analyze the concentration of gases for the purpose of discovering the purity of the gas inside the multiplace hyperbaric chamber. Gas analyzers can detect the presence and purity of oxygen, air, and carbon dioxide. Some gas analyzers are portable and some are wall mounted or panel mounted. An area of elevated oxygen inside a multiplace chamber is a high risk for a fire. If the air inside the chamber is continuously circulated, a local area of concentrated oxygen will not be allowed to form. National Fire Protection Association Health Care Facilities Code 99 (NFPA 99) requires a minimum vent of three actual cubic feet per minute) for each person not on a mask or hood equipped with an overboard dump. The ignition temperature levels of flammable materials drop when the oxygen concentration exceeds 23.5%. This is why multiplace chamber oxygen levels must not exceed 23.5% per NFPA 99.

Critical need for oxygen purity in a gas supply system

Oxygen gas purity is not only critical for proper patient treatment, but it is also critical for keeping the patient and staff safe in their environment. Inside a multiplace chamber, the oxygen content must be no greater than 23.5%, or there is risk of fire. Carbon dioxide levels must be kept below 2.5% by volume at a depth of 33 fsw, or 2 atmospheres absolute. If there is not a proper overboard dump in place, a carbon dioxide scrubber may be installed. The Sodasorb (carbon dioxide absorbent) inside a scrubber filters the air as it passes through. This scrubber may be a stand-alone unit. The carbon dioxide levels inside a hood or mask must be kept below 0.005%. The higher the carbon dioxide level, the greater the chance of an oxygen-toxicity seizure. The goal of 100% oxygen delivered to the patient is the sole purpose of the hyperbaric treatment, so the oxygen content must be pure.

Risks associated with a contaminated gas line

Gas lines carry 100% oxygen and must not be contaminated in any way. Depending on what the gas line may be contaminated with, there is risk of oxygen toxicity by onloading of carbon dioxide. If the air compressor of a multiplace chamber is compromised in any way, it could pose a risk to the patient and the staff. If the air quality going into the air compressor is contaminated, the air quality of the chamber atmosphere will be contaminated. Coordinate with hospital or facility staff to ensure exhausts and other possible contaminants are not installed or in operation near or around the compressor. The best source for a contaminate detector is the human nose. Be sure to inspect the air quality daily, and to analyze the oxygen content frequently as policy dictates.

Importance of filtering the gas line in the supply system

Solid contaminates and particles of metal, polytetrafluoroethylene (the film used in sealing pipe threads), or carbon may be present at the air intake of the compressor. It is important to have a filtration system in place to filter out these contaminates. The compressor itself may even generate these contaminates and particles. For this reason, the filtration system must be inspected frequently. For oxygen lines, fittings, valves, regulators, and pressure gauges that are required to pass high pressure and high percentages of oxygen, they must be cleaned for oxygen service and must be deemed "O_2 safe." All gas lines, valves, and regulators for oxygen use only must be marked accordingly with clear, readable, colored signage.

Process for carbon dioxide analysis

Inside a multiplace chamber, the levels of carbon dioxide must be measured using a gas analyzer per the National Fire Protection Association Health Care Facilities Code 99 (NFPA 99). When the chamber is on the surface, the carbon dioxide (CO_2) levels must be no greater than 5% volume. As the depth of the chamber increases, the safe CO_2 level decreases. At two atmospheres absolute, or 33 feet of seawater, the safe CO_2 partial pressure is 2.5% of the volume. The flow of masks and hoods for oxygen breathing should be set to an efficient amount to prevent CO_2 buildup greater than 0.005%. A good, tight seal on masks and hoods will help to prevent higher than normal CO_2 levels. High CO_2 levels put patients at risk for an oxygen-toxicity seizure.

Process for oxygen analysis

The oxygen concentration inside a multiplace chamber must be no greater than 23.5%, according to the National Fire Protection Association Health Care Facilities Code 99 (NFPA 99). An oxygen level above 23.5% poses a great risk of fire. A typical oxygen analyzer uses a sensor that generates an electrical current when introduced to an oxygen environment. The gas analyzer must be calibrated daily. The sensor has a six-month expiration time because it degenerates after each use. There must be a sample flow rate consistent with the flow rate in the chamber passing across the sensor for the data to be accurate. Possible courses of actions to take when the oxygen level raises are to increase chamber vent rate or the inside tender searches for the oxygen leak source, which may be a loose hood connection, torn hood, or torn neck ring. The overboard dump system may need to be reviewed. The oxygen pipe fittings may be leaking, or there could be a faulty regulator. If troubleshooting the reason for high oxygen detection fails, the dive should be aborted.

Calibrating gas analyzers

Gas analyzers may be calibrated separately or together, depending on the type and gas analyzed. Oxygen gas content/percentage should be constantly monitored in a multiplace chamber. The oxygen gas analyzer is calibrated to 20.9% when sampling ambient air. It should be connected to the chamber air sample port, and it should be equipped with audio and visual alarms for unsafe oxygen levels. According to the National Fire Protection

Association Health Care Facilities Code 99 (NFPA 99), the oxygen percentage of the air in the multiplace chamber should be no greater than 23.5%. Fuel cell or paramagnetic oxygen analyzers are most often used to monitor the oxygen percentages of both the hyperbaric chamber and the patient hoods. These do not require recalibration between reading air and pure oxygen once they have been calibrated. Some systems may use one analyzer to monitor O_2, CO_2, and CO from the air. Usually, a gas mixture sample may be used to calibrate these types of analyzers.

Confirming calibration when delivering multiple gases during hyperbaric operations

Calibration of gas analyzers may be confirmed by using the calibrated analyzer to sample a premixed gas cylinder. Or the facility may have multiple gas analyzers, and they may be used to confirm calibration against each other. The premixed sample gas cylinder must be an accurate sampling of the gas being analyzed inside the chamber. The calibration gas flow across the sensor must be at a consistent rate. Likewise, the chamber gas flow rate should be equal to the calibration gas flow rate. If they are not consistent together, the chamber gas percentage reading will not be accurate, and it may lead the chamber operator to realize a false high oxygen reading.

Indications and treatment of nitrogen narcosis

Divers and inside tenders for multiplace chambers may fall victim to nitrogen narcosis if they dive deeper than a depth of 100 feet on air. The symptoms of nitrogen narcosis are similar to the symptoms of a drug-induced state. The diver may have trouble accomplishing simple tasks and may not be able to think clearly. The “narced-out” diver will hyperventilate and take on too much carbon dioxide, eventually passing out. The treatment for nitrogen narcosis is simple; either decompress the diver to a depth of less than 100 feet or switch the diving gas to 100% oxygen or a mixture thereof.

Air breaks for patients during a hyperbaric treatment

Hyperbaric oxygen treatments deeper than 2 atmospheres absolute (ATA) require the patient to take air breaks. If the patient is diving at 2 ATA, but is having multiple treatments a day, he/she is required to take air breaks. Air breaks can be customized by a hyperbaric physician’s order depending on the indication the patient is diving for. The typical air break protocol for a patient diving at 2.5 ATA is 15 minutes to travel to the treatment depth, 30 minutes at depth, followed by a 5-minute air break, and then another 30 minutes of oxygen at depth followed by a second 5-minute air break. Finally, the patient breathes 30 more minutes of oxygen before decompressing to the surface for 15 minutes. Examples of indications with air breaks are radiation injuries, carbon monoxide poisoning, and gas gangrene.

Equipment for monitoring the chamber for depth, temperature, and humidity

For hyperbaric chambers, the monitoring process is either done manually or electronically. Manual chambers are monitored by the use of pressure gauges. The pressure going to the hyperbaric chamber is diverted into the pressure gauges, causing the needle to move concurrent with the pressure in the chamber. The electronically monitored chamber uses an electronic control module for pressure control and temperature monitoring. The pressure from the chamber is routed by tubes to the electronic control module, which feeds information to the electronic console. The manual chamber console monitors the pressure and rate of pressure, whereas the electronic chamber console can monitor the pressure, rate of pressure, and temperature.

Portable vs. panel-mounted analysis equipment

The portable oxygen gas analyzer is very simple to use and to calibrate. The best advantage of the portable analyzer is that it may be moved to analyze pockets of gas in hard-to-access areas of the multiplace hyperbaric chamber. The sensor on this analyzer degenerates with every use, and it may need to be replaced every six months. To calibrate, uncover the sensor and set it to 20.9%. The panel-mounted gas analyzer is more complex. The best advantage of the panel-mounted analyzer is that it may analyze multiple gases at the same time. This analyzer also requires daily calibration by using a special mixture of calibration gas. The sample gas and the sample flow rate must be the same sampling as that inside the chamber.

Causes of gas stratification

Gas stratification is the movement of gases from one elevation to another, depending on the weight of the gases and the absence of air movement. For example, a balloon filled with helium will rise, while a balloon filled with air will fall. A dense gas such as carbon dioxide will fall to a lower elevation in a tank or chamber. If there is a heliox gas mixture, the helium will rise to the top of the chamber. Gas stratification is usually not relevant to most gas-monitoring situations because of the ventilations that occur. That is why it is important to vent the chamber at regular intervals. When entering a sealed, enclosed space that has had no or little air movement, such as a multiplace hyperbaric chamber, it is important to follow the rules and regulations of confined spaces. Stagnant pockets of gas, no matter the cause, may be damaging, or even deadly.

Maintaing records for the hyperbaric delivery system

Incremental records should be maintained for each chamber including all daily logs and checklists, weekly preventative maintenance checklists, and monthly inspection and maintenance checklists for up to two years. The chamber's history records are to be kept for the life of the chamber such as the 510(k) Summary of Safety and Effectiveness, which documents the intended use, performance standards, approved indications, and a device description. The 510(k) is required and reviewed by the Food and Drug Administration. Annual maintenance reports should be provided by an approved chamber service company, usually the manufacturer. Chamber installation documentation includes the inspection certificate, the installing technician certification, the certification of installment and any preinstallment forms such as American Society of Mechanical Engineers and pressure vessels for human occupancy data reports. Lastly, all maintenance and repair logs should be retained.

Purpose of a gas status board and how it is used

Gas status boards are maintained by the hyperbaric technologist or the hyperbaric safety director. The purpose of the gas status board is to keep a running status of current gas mixtures and gas reserves. The technologist may also use the gas status board to keep a daily record of the primary and secondary liquid oxygen tank supplies. The air cylinder supply levels should be recorded daily as well as the number of oxygen tanks with their supply pressures. The gas status board should also reflect the cylinder for calibration mixture and its specific gas mixture supply. As the gas supply changes between dives in the multiplace chamber and other procedures for patient use, the gas status board should be updated.

Chamber Operations and Environment

Sequential steps for operating a monoplace hyperbaric chamber

The procedures to operate a monoplace hyperbaric chamber are as follows: All chamber predive checklist items must be completed. Verify the presence of the oxygen supply pressure. The chamber door must be closed and locked. The master control knob must be turned to the "on" position. Gas will start to flow and the chamber will compress to an idle pressure, usually 1.5psig. For chambers with an electronic panel, the electronic control system will automatically turn on self-test. Make sure that all segments of the display are activated. An audible alarm may also sound. If there is a patient inside the chamber, make sure he or she is briefed on the sounds to expect during the treatment. The chamber will indicate pressurization at this time. The intercom system will automatically come on with certain chamber types, although some chambers have a separate intercom switch. The rate set knob must be set to the desired rate of compression. Use the pressure set knob to set the chamber pressure to the treatment depth. The chamber will reach and remain at the treatment depth until a new set pressure is entered. When the treatment is complete, turn the pressure set knob down to idle pressure, or zero, depending on chamber type. After idle pressure is reached, turn the master control knob to the "off" position, wait until the chamber is completely depressurized, and unlock and open the chamber door.

Inside tender's role in the multiplace chamber

Hyperbaric treatments involving a multiplace chamber require a chamber attendant, also known as an inside tender. The inside tender is accountable for all operations within the multiplace chamber and should be familiar with all of the signs and symptoms of pressure-related issues and all treatment protocols. He or she is also responsible for communicating with medical personnel outside of the chamber, taking vital signs as needed, administering oxygen as required, constant patient observation, and providing general assistance. If the patients are anxious inside of the chamber, it is the tender's job to calm and reassure them. The tender should hold the oxygen mask to the patient's face versus strapping it on in case of oxygen-toxicity seizures. The inside tender should also keep track of his or her own dive log and profile, and he or she should intermittently breathe 100% oxygen as required to avoid nitrogen narcosis.

Weekly system checks and user maintenance needed for an active hyperbaric chamber

The weekly monoplace hyperbaric chamber checks include multiple steps. First, complete the daily startup checklist. Then, prepare fresh disinfection/cleaning solution as required. Next, clean the interior and exterior of the chamber as well as the exhaust filter. In a monoplace chamber, the exhaust filter may be detached using a Phillips-head screwdriver, soak the filter in water, and blow it clean using pressurized air. Clean the gurney and sled, as well as the mattress, pillows, and positioning pads. Then, pressurize the chamber to 2 atmospheres absolute (ATA). Verify the calibration and operation of the set and chamber pressure gauges. Record the minimum and maximum purge/ventilation flow rates depending on the chamber type. Wait 12 minutes and record the minimum and maximum plateau flow rates. Next, pressurize the chamber to 3 ATA and check for leaks. Depressurize the chamber using the emergency vent/exhaust button, and record the time: It must be less than or equal to 2 minutes. Verify that the safety lock pin disengages at pressures lower than 1 psig. Verify chamber depressurization. Test the facility ground (it must be less than 1 ohm), and test the patient ground cord (the range is from 0.950 to 1.050 M ohm). Inspect the emergency smoke mask and check its expiration date. Inspect the chamber exterior exhaust monthly. Finally, complete the daily shutdown checklist.

Performing predive checks and user maintenance before operating the hyperbaric chamber

The predive checks start with checking and recording the oxygen supply levels. The primary and secondary tanks are usually located outside of the facility. The air supply tanks are usually next to the chambers. If not, they can be found in a utility closet close enough to route the lines to the chambers. Chamber inspection involves carefully studying the acrylic for scratches outside and inside. Buff out any scratches in a timely manner using an approved scratch remover. The door lock and locking pin should be operated daily before patient use by running up the chamber to idle pressure; the gauges, knobs, and communication device may also be checked at this time. The door gasket may be damaged from use. It is best to keep a spare gasket on hand for timely replacement. The supply and exhaust hoses, grounding cable, and other connections should be secure. Become familiar with these attachments and their purpose for future troubleshooting. Be sure the stretcher operates correctly by attaching a sled to a gurney and locking and unlocking the stretcher. Be sure the emergency breathing device is present and has not expired.

Performing postdive checks and user maintenance after operating hyperbaric chamber

The postdive checks must be performed by the technologist daily and after the last chamber treatment. Always check to make sure the master control is in the "off" position. The oxygen valve is usually located on the wall in the back of the chamber. Be sure to close the oxygen valve. Close the air valve as well, and bleed the remaining air from the lines. The chamber must be thoroughly cleaned if it is dirty and especially if a patient with an infectious disease has had a chamber treatment. The stretcher must be cleaned after every patient and prepared with fresh linens. To keep the sled and linens fresh, place the sled inside the chamber. Keep the chamber covered at night to keep dust away and to keep it secure.

Predive checks using specific checklists for the hyperbaric chamber

Predive checks should be performed daily using a specific checklist. The checklist should be in hand and followed precisely. Record the primary and secondary oxygen supplies. Inspect the chamber acrylic exterior. Inspect the chamber door locking mechanism. Inspect the chamber gurney and sled, and remove them from the chamber. Ensure that the gurney wheels lock and that the stretcher latches. Inspect the integrity of the chamber door gasket. Inspect the chamber acrylic interior. Inspect the supply and exhaust hoses. Inspect the chamber ground cable and connections. Inspect the power supply cables and connections. Slowly open the oxygen supply valve. Inspect the air hose and connections. Slowly open the air supply valve and record the pressure (minimum 500 psig). Inspect the pressure gauge faces, flowmeter, and indicator lenses and the control, communication, and flow knobs. Verify communication functions. Close and lock the chamber door. Turn the master valve on and verify that the locking pin engages; then turn the master valve off. Check for the presence of the staff emergency breathing mask. Inspect the patient grounding cord. Lastly, ensure that the source selector is set to oxygen, if installed.

Postdive checks using specific checklists for the hyperbaric chamber

Postdive checks should be performed daily when the last dive is completed using a specific checklist. The checklist should be in hand, and it should be followed precisely. First, ensure that the master valve is in the "off" position. Close the oxygen supply valve. Close the air supply valve, and bleed the air from the line to zero. Verify that the interior and exterior of the chamber are clean. Clean and prepare the gurney for the next day. Place the clean sled inside the chamber. Secure the chamber door. Lastly, cover the chamber. It is easy to get complacent regarding these checklists, especially if they are daily. It is very important to stay on point and routinely complete these checks. If just one item is missed, it could mean jeopardizing the safety of the entire hyperbaric facility. Physicians, nurses, and patients rely on the hyperbaric technologist to keep safety as the number-one priority.

Types of medical locks and ancillary safety devices and their application

A multiplace hyperbaric chamber may incorporate a medical lock as well as a primary lock compartment and a main compartment. The primary lock compartment is used for locking tenders and equipment into and out of a pressurized chamber. A medical lock is used for locking medications and other equipment into and out of the chamber. A medical lock may be used as opposed to a primary lock because it is smaller in size and easier to pressurize to depth. Medical locks are typically 12 inches square, and the doors may be of single-handed operation. Other ancillary equipment includes handlines for fire safety, masks for inside tenders breathing oxygen, a carbon monoxide scrubber, patient hoods, beds, and chairs. The equipment for inside hyperbaric chamber use should be specialized materials/equipment for high-oxygen-concentration and pressurized environments.

Recommended equipment for optimal chamber pressurization

For a multiplace hyperbaric chamber, the needed equipment for pressurization is an air compressor. The air compressor is high pressure (around 2000 psi), and it is lubricated with oil specified for use for high temperatures. If proper maintenance of the compressor is not completed, the temperatures inside the compressor may rise to a point of oxidizing the lubrication oil into carbon monoxide gas. A filter system including a Hopcalite catalyst may be fitted onto the compressor to convert the carbon monoxide gas into carbon dioxide gas. The system must be cleaned and maintained in order to prevent breakdown or possible explosion. The monoplace chamber is pressurized by a high-pressure oxygen feed from a liquid oxygen system. The high pressure is reduced by regulators along the gas lines.

Recommended fire suppression system to meet regulatory requirements

According to the NFPA 99, a fire suppression system is required for multiplace chambers. The fire suppression system that is installed in the multiplace chamber consists of an independently supplied handline and a deluge-type water-spray system. These two systems are separate so that if one fails, the other will not be affected. The fire suppression system controls will be located on the chamber operator's console. When either the handline or deluge system is activated, the ungrounded electrical components are automatically disconnected, audio and visual alarms sound, and emergency lighting is activated. If a deluge system is installed in more than one area of the chamber, both systems will be able to act together or separately. Water is discharged from the deluge system nozzle within 3 seconds of activation. The nozzle spray will be on average 2 gal/ft^2. Two handlines will be strategically located within the compartment and will operate at 5 gal/ft^2.

Proper care and maintenance of acrylic viewports/cylinders

The acrylic surface is extremely susceptible to scratching, so vigilance is needed when caring for viewports. Never allow anyone to lean on the chamber. When cleaning the acrylic, avoid abrasion of the surface. Do not allow liquids or solvents to come into contact with the acrylic surface. Clean up any spills as soon as possible. Use a lint-free, 100% cotton cloth moistened with water to remove dust from the acrylic. To wash the acrylic window, use a soft cloth made with 100% cotton and moistened with a mild detergent solution. Rinse and dry with a soft 100% cotton cloth. Do not use any alcohol- or oil-based substances on the acrylic window. If water accumulates in the bottom of the chamber, it might drain into and contaminate the supply or exhaust piping. Keep the acrylic in pristine condition for a high level of patient comfort.

Implications of crazing on the chamber acrylic

The definition of crazing is an extended network of cracking that may spread under the surface of the acrylic or run through the plastic; it presents as microcracks. Crazing on the surface of the acrylic is usually from a type of stress called tensile stress. The conditions for the development of stress crazing are acrylic sheet stress and the introduction of an aggressive liquid or solvent. Both of these conditions must be met in order to cause crazing. Cleaning agents or solvent used on the chamber acrylic must be dried as soon as possible to prevent chemical harm to the surface. During the manufacturing process, the acrylic sheet may undergo what is called "cold forming." A polarized light may be used to detect the presence of cold forming. Stress may also occur during the cooling phase after the acrylic is formed and reinforced with a fiberglass mixture. Lastly, uneven structure support of the finished part may result in additional stress. Daily inspections of the acrylic are required before pressurization.

Approaches to monitoring gases breathed by patients and/or tenders

The gases that are breathed in by the patients or the inside tenders must be monitored to ensure overall quality and medical and fire safety and that the gases for chamber pressurization meet or exceed the standard for grade D air. Air samples may be taken once a month and when work is done on the compressor. The air samples must be taken at the air intakes and the compressor discharge line. Multiplace and monoplace chambers usually operate with a constant vent, ensuring that the carbon dioxide is continuously dumped and fresh oxygen or air is piped in. The percentages of oxygen and carbon dioxide may also be monitored by use of a gas analyzer in some chambers. Ensure that the gas analyzers are calibrated with either a premixed calibration gas or by sources of 21% and 100% oxygen.

Types of sampling conducted when monitoring external gas quality

Air and oxygen used in multiplace and monoplace chambers must be periodically sampled for gas purity. The oxygen that derives its source from the hospital's liquid oxygen (LOX) system is typically monitored and sampled by the outside company that delivers the LOX.

Each time the LOX is delivered, the hospital safety staff and the hyperbaric technologist should receive a certificate of gas purity that is equal to or greater than 99.5%. The air that is used for multiplace hyperbaric chamber pressurization must be sampled every 30 days and sent to a laboratory where it is analyzed using a mass spectrometer and/or a gas chromatograph. Air samples are analyzed for total hydrocarbons, nitrous oxides, carbon monoxide, carbon dioxide and oxygen, nitrogen, and moisture content. Air samples may also be taken when work is done to the compressor. Air samples must be taken at the intake and at the discharge of the compressor.

Delivering oxygen to patients within a multiplace chamber via a hood

In the multiplace hyperbaric chamber, a patient may receive 100% oxygen through a hood device. This is the most common method for this type of chamber. A top and a neck dam are the two basic components of the hood. The top is made up of a cylinder-shaped plastic tent attached at the bottom to a ring. The neck dam is made of latex that encircles the neck and is attached to a mounting ring. This mounting ring corresponds to the ring on the hood, and the two may be easily attached and detached. Before the use of the neck dam, the hood was attached to the patient by taping it directly to the skin. The supply and exhaust ports may or may not be incorporated into the neck dam, depending on the manufacturer. Patients tend to prefer the hood to the mask because it is less constrictive.

Delivering oxygen to patients within a hyperbaric chamber via a mask

A mask may be used in a monoplace and in a multiplace chamber. There are two types of masks used currently: a demand mask and a free-flow mask. A demand mask has a one-way valve that uses the pressure of the patient's inhalation to deliver oxygen on demand. The demand mask is made up of a plastic mask piece that covers the mouth and the nose, a regulator with an attached valve and valve cover, and a filter. This assembly attaches to a hose and then a port with a quarter-turn ball valve (multiplace only) inside the chamber. The demand mask assembly must be cleaned between patient uses. The free-flow mask is a disposable, nonrebreather mask (monoplace only) attached to a port in the chamber.

Devices used inside the multiplace chamber that deliver breathing gases via masks or hoods

Inside the multiplace hyperbaric chamber, regulators are used to deliver breathing gases to hoods and masks. The high-pressure gas in a cylinder or a liquid oxygen converter is too high to use in clinical practice and needs to be regulated to a lower usable pressure. Specific regulators are used for specific gases, and they are designed to handle high and low pressures. Pressure reduction may be accomplished by a one- or two-stage regulator. The one-stage regulator reduces high pressure (2000 psi) down to a working pressure (40 to 70 psi), and then on to a flowmeter. Flowmeters directly control breathing gases and have a maximum inlet pressure of 100 psi. A two-stage regulator reduces the high pressure to a medium pressure to possibly be distributed to multiple sources, and then it is further reduced to a low working pressure as needed.

Compression and decompression operating procedures for air or gas embolism

Air or gas embolism (AGE) and decompression sickness are typically treated in a recompression chamber with the *U.S. Navy Diving Manual* tables. Both indications are treated with treatment tables 5 and 6 at 60 feet of seawater (fsw) if the symptoms are relieved. If the symptoms are not relieved, the patient is then taken down to 165 fsw for a treatment table 6A. Type I decompression sickness is treated with table 5 at 60 fsw. If there is no relief, the treatment becomes a table 6. Decompression sickness type II and AGE are treated with treatment table 6 to begin with. The treatment becomes a table 6A if there has been no relief of symptoms on table 6.

Diagnostic indicators

Carbon monoxide and cyanide poisoning diagnostic indicators

The treatment protocol for carbon monoxide and cyanide poisoning is hyperbaric oxygen. Patients with this diagnosis should receive hyperbaric oxygen therapy within 24 hours of exposure. For the first hyperbaric chamber treatment, the patient should be pressurized to 3 atmospheres absolute (ATA) in 15 minutes. The patient should be at pressure for 25 minutes and then take a 5-minute air break. Then, the technologist should repeat the 25 minutes of oxygen followed by 5 minutes of air. The patient is then traveled to 2 ATA where he or she will have two 30-minute oxygen periods with a 5-minute air break in between. The patient is then depressurized over 15 minutes. For the next two chamber treatments, the patient is pressurized to 2 ATA for three 30-minute periods of oxygen breathing with 5-minute air breaks in between. These treatments must be separated by a 4-hour surface time.

Clostridial myonecrosis diagnostic indicators

The treatment protocol for gas gangrene is hyperbaric oxygen therapy. The treatment schedule should be followed closely for this indication, and treatment should commence within the first 24 hours of diagnosis. The patient is pressurized to a depth of 3 atmospheres absolute (ATA) for 90 minutes while breathing 100% oxygen. This 90-minute interval is usually split into three 25-minute periods with a 5-minute air break in between, or two 45-minute intervals with a 5-minute air break between. Some facilities, depending on their policies, will treat the patient at 2.5 ATA instead. The first three hyperbaric oxygen treatments should be within the first 24 hours with an interval of 4 hours between treatments. Some seriously ill patients will require only 2 hours between the first two treatments.

Diabetic foot ulcer diagnostic indicators

A diabetic foot ulcer (DFU) is a chronic wound with bacterial organisms that have colonized. Hyperbaric oxygen therapy treats DFUs by reversing the hypoxia in the local tissue and killing the bacterial organisms that are causing the infection. Through hyperbaric oxygen therapy (HBOT), the increased tissue oxygenation increases the formation of free radicals, which kill bacterial organisms as an antibacterial agent. To qualify for HBOT treatments, the patient must be a diabetic with a Wagner III grade wound on a lower extremity. The wound must not show signs of improvement for at least 30 days. HBOT must be used in conjunction with revascularization, wound care, and glucose and nutritional control. DFUs are typically treated at 2 atmospheres absolute for 90 minutes while breathing 100% oxygen with no air breaks. The treatments are five days a week for a duration of 20 to 30 treatments.

Chronic osteomyelitis (refractory) diagnostic indicators

Hyperbaric oxygen therapy when used in conjunction with antibiotics is indicated for the management of chronic refractory osteomyelitis, secondary to surgery. The recommended treatment course for this diagnosis is 20 to 40 treatments inside a hyperbaric chamber at one treatment per day. The patient is pressurized to 2 atmospheres absolute for 90 minutes while breathing 100% oxygen. No air breaks are required at this pressure unless the patient is predisposed to seizure activity. The pretreatment course recommendation prior to surgery is at least 10 treatments. The patient must complete the entire course of treatments in order to have optimal wound healing through oxygenation.

Necrotizing soft-tissue infections diagnostic indicators

An adjunctive treatment protocol for necrotizing soft tissue infections (necrotizing fasciitis) is hyperbaric oxygen therapy (HBOT) along with a course of antibiotics. HBOT treatments are typically started after the first surgical debridement. The patient should receive three treatments within the first 24 hours with intervals of 4 hours between treatments. The patient is pressurized to 3 atmospheres absolute for 90 minutes while breathing 100% oxygen. This 90-minute period may be broken up into two 45-minute intervals with a 5-minute air break in between or three 25-minute intervals with 5-minute air breaks between them. The treatments are continued twice a day after day one if improvement is seen. The full treatment course is 10 to 15 days.

Delayed radiation injuries (soft-tissue and bony necrosis) diagnostic indicator

Hyperbaric oxygen therapy (HBOT)is used as an adjunctive treatment secondary to surgery. Surgery for radiation injuries should be performed after 20 treatments in a hyperbaric chamber has been completed, with the patient receiving 10 more treatments postsurgery. The HBOT protocol for a radiation injury is pressurization to 2.5 atmospheres absolute (ATA) for 90 minutes while breathing 100% oxygen with two 5-minute air breaks. Some clinics only pressurize patients to 2 ATA. In that case, the patient should be at depth for 120 minutes. Radiation injuries have a better response at 3 ATA, but this depth is potentially too toxic for multiple treatments. All patients at depth should be watched closely for signs of oxygen toxicity, but especially patients at a depth deeper than 2 ATA. Two sessions of HBOT per day have been suggested, but the protocol has not been proven or tested and may not be clinically practical.

Intracranial abscess diagnostic indicators

Hyperbaric oxygen therapy (HBOT) used along with antibiotics is an adjunctive therapy to an intracranial abscess, secondary to surgery. HBOT is approved for use in the following situations: when the patient has no surgical response, anaerobic or mixed pathogens are present, multiple abscesses are present, in a compromised host, or when surgery is contraindicated. The HBOT protocol for this diagnosis is early administration at 2.5 atmospheres absolute for 90 minutes while breathing 100% oxygen. This 90-minute period may be broken up by two 45-minute periods with a 5-minute air break in between, or three 25-minute periods with 5-minute air breaks between them. Two treatments per day are recommended. The number of treatments is determined on an individual basis.

Exceptional blood loss anemia diagnostic indicators

For the case of extreme anemia, hyperbaric oxygen therapy (HBOT) is indicated to oxygenate the patient enough until he or she can produce hemoglobin sufficient to meet the physiologic demands for basic oxygen delivery in the body. The HBOT treatments should be initiated as soon after the diagnosis as possible. For the first treatment, the patient is pressurized to 3 atmospheres absolute (ATA) for 30 minutes while breathing 100% oxygen with a 5-minute air break. The patient then travels to 2 ATA for 90 minutes at 100% oxygen. This 90 minutes is split up into three 30-minute intervals with two 5-minute air breaks in between segments. For extreme cases, a surface interval of only one hour is required before the next 90-minute treatment at depth.

Ischemia/reperfusion diagnostic indicators

Ischemia/reperfusion (IR) injuries are typical of patients with a high-energy trauma or an amputated body part. Any time a part of the body is subjected to prolonged periods of ischemia followed by sudden reperfusion, an accelerated microcirculatory injury could take place and cell death may occur. Hyperbaric oxygen therapy (HBOT) for IR injuries has been considered to be controversial in the past, but subsequent animal testing has proven that hyperoxygenation of an ischemic injury that has been recently reperfused is beneficial to the wound. Hyperbaric oxygen actually improves skin flaps and grafts after an IR injury. The primary treatment for this type of injury is surgery to restore blood flow, and the secondary treatment is HBOT to make the blood flow effective. HBOT must initiate as soon as possible after surgery, preferably within one hour. Pressurization at 2.5 ATA for 90 minutes while breathing 100% oxygen with two 5-minute air breaks is the recommended treatment.

Crush injury/compartment syndrome diagnostic indicators

The management of crush injuries and compartment syndrome may be accomplished through the adjunctive use of hyperbaric oxygen therapy (HBOT). HBOT is approved for maintaining tissue viability and facilitating healing and durable effects. Transcutaneous oxygen measurements are useful in determining the viability of tissue throughout the course of treatments. HBOT is recommended to commence as early as possible from the first sign of injury, usually within 4 to 6 hours. The amount of treatments depends on the desired outcome of this modality. HBOT treatments are typically given at 2 atmospheres absolute (ATA) for 90 minutes while breathing 100% oxygen and no air breaks. An alternate method is to pressurize the patient to 2.5 ATA for 90 minutes of 100% oxygen with two 5-minute air breaks.

Compromised grafts and flaps diagnostic indicators

HBOT is indicated for compromised skin flaps and grafts as an adjunctive treatment secondary to surgery. Hyperbaric treatments are typically given at 2.5 atmospheres absolute (ATA) for 90 minutes while breathing 100% oxygen with two 5-minute air breaks, or 2 ATA for 120 minutes while breathing 100% oxygen. One treatment per day for five days a week is recommended, for a total of 20 to 30 treatments. A utilization review is required after 20 treatments to determine the efficacy of the HBO therapy. An in-chamber transcutaneous oxygen measurement (TCOM) or a room-air TCOM may be used for collecting evidence during the review. HBOT can preserve tissues that are not healing and are compromised. HBOT delivers oxygen to these tissues, increasing their oxygen tensions and inducing wound healing by collagen synthesis and fibroblast development. The vasoconstrictive properties of HBOT improve blood circulation to the wound.

Acute thermal burn injury indicator

Hyperbaric oxygen therapy (HBOT) is an adjunctive treatment for thermal burns. HBOT for acute thermal burn injury is held as a controversial therapy because it is either too dangerous or too expensive, but nevertheless, it has been shown to be a very effective treatment for this type of injury. The leading cause of death from thermal burns is infection. HBOT fights infection with its antibacterial processes. Edema is also a factor in thermal burns, and hyperbaric oxygen vasoconstricts the blood vessels and lessens edema in the tissues. Patients selected for HBOT typically have more than 20% thermal burns of the total body surface, either partial thickness or full thickness and in specific areas. The treatment protocol of hyperbaric oxygen therapy for thermal burn injuries is 2 ATA for 90 minutes with no air breaks, twice a day.

Off-label disorders

The off-label use of hyperbaric oxygen therapy is controversial and has raised ethical concerns. Some public facilities that advertise for off-label uses do not have properly credentialed medical staff or specialized physician supervision and may not be strictly following Food and Drug Administration (FDA) regulations. Patients and family members could be taken advantage of financially and may not have informed consent. Some facilities, for example, will treat off-label conditions at 1.3 atmospheres absolute (ATA) with air, which is the same as receiving 27% oxygen at sea level, or treatments at 1.3 ATA with 24% oxygen, which is only 31% oxygen at sea level. Some conditions, such as femoral head necrosis, may be treated at 2 to 2.5 ATA for 90 minutes, but patients must typically receive 100 treatments in order to achieve their healing goals. In some of these cases, hyperbaric oxygen therapy has been shown to work; however, off-label conditions are not FDA approved due to a lack of controlled clinical trials and evidence, and these treatments are not covered by insurance.

Hardware components of the breathing gas system

Cylinders, gas lines, fittings, pressure gauges, valves, and regulators are essential to the gas breathing system. The cylinder is used for gas cylinders and is designed according to the amount of gas needed. Gas lines are designed to carry different amounts of pressure, and they may be thick-walled for high pressure or thin-walled for low pressure. Copper tubing is typically used for hyperbaric gases. Gas lines must be secured at regular intervals and marked for directional flow and gas identification. Fittings may be attached to tubing or equipment by brazing or compression, depending on the pressure and tube size. All fittings must be leak tested and gas compatible. All oxygen gas hardware needs to be cleaned for oxygen service before use. Pressure gauges must be certified and rated for the specific gas in the system. Valves turn the system on and off, and they control excessive pressures and flow direction. Regulators are used for pressure reduction.

Key points in the history of hyperbarics

Important developments throughout the history of hyperbarics include: the relation between pressure and volume (Boyle, 1660), the discovery of oxygen (Priestley, 1774), the understanding of the toxic effects of oxygen (Seguin & Lavoisier, 1789), the first book on oxygen therapy (Beddoes & Watt, 1796), the discovery of central nervous system oxygen toxicity (Bert, 1878), decompression schedules (Haldane, 1905), a treatment for decompression sickness (Behnke & Shaw,1937), radiation treatments (Churchill-Davidson et al., 1955), the publication: *Life Without Blood* (Boerema, 1960), hyperbaric oxygen therapy evidence of efficacy in wounds (1960–1970), the formation and development of the Undersea and Hyperbaric Medical Society (1967) and the Divers Alert Network (1980), and finally, the formation of the International Society of Hyperbaric Medicine (1988).

Required maintenance for medical gas tanks, lines, and fittings

Gas lines for gas breathing systems typically are made from copper tubing (type K or L seamless copper). If a gas line made from copper tubing has dents, scratches, or unintentional bends, then replacement is required immediately. When copper tubing is bent, it should have a smooth radial curve so as not to be overstressed. Fittings and gas lines should be oxygen cleaned if used for oxygen breathing purposes. Cylinders may have a valve that will not turn, or they may leak gas when the valve is closed. These cylinders will require maintenance before use. Do not expose cylinders to high temperatures because the increased pressure may cause the cylinder to explode. If the cylinder does not have a label, do not use it. All cylinders must be hydrostatically tested every 5 or 10 years. The test date is stamped on the cylinder.

Preventing gas leaks using proper fittings and thread forms

Gas leaks can be prevented when installing gas lines and fittings. For oxygen tubing and fittings, nitrogen is pressure leak tested using a solution of soap and water at the fitting attachment points. Ensure the cleanliness of the tubing and fittings by removing any residue made by the leak test solution with a clean cloth. A leak-tight seal should be provided on the fitting thread forms. A sealant may be used on the male fittings. Thread-seal tape (polytetrafluoroethylene) is the most common sealant type used for gas breathing systems. Thread-seal tape is most useful because it provides a sealant and a lubricant. The tape should be fitted around the threads of the male fitting, but not past the first thread. Other products may be used for sealant; however, any product that is used must be compatible with gas breathing systems.

Monitoring and routine maintenance of the chamber life support system

Hyperbaric chambers are pressure vessels into which human beings may be placed for treatment. The vessel is pressurized with either air (multiplace) or oxygen (monoplace), and persons inside may breathe the atmosphere or breathe through a mask. These systems are monitored by a gas selection valve on the chamber console, a quarter-turn ball valve on the chamber gas intake line, and/or use of a gas analyzer. These systems are maintained by use of a regular maintenance routine, which includes daily, weekly, monthly, quarterly, and annual inspections. Fire safety equipment may be installed inside and outside the chamber. This equipment includes handlines, waterspray deluge systems, water tanks, and an emergency exhaust/vent button on the chamber console.

Classification of gas cylinders

Cylinders may be classified by color, size, and air letter grade. These classifications are specified by the Compressed Gas Association. Air letter grades D, E, and N are approved for use in gas breathing systems. Grade D air is approved for use in industrial breathing systems. Grade E air is used for scuba diving. Grade N air is used for medical gases. Cylinder sizes used for hyperbaric purposes are size H and size E. Size H cylinders have 2000–3000 psi, and hold 244 cubic feet of gas. Size E cylinders have 2000 psi and hold about 660 liters of oxygen. Size H cylinders are usually backup high-pressure tanks, and they are typically stationary. Size E cylinders are very mobile and are used mostly for transporting patients who need oxygen. The cylinder colors we use in hyperbaric applications are yellow for air; green for oxygen; and there are some uses for nitrogen, which is black in color.

Safety guideline "do's" to be followed for gas cylinders

For safety reasons, there some guidelines to follow for gas cylinders. The Compressed Gas Association has listed regulations on using and storing cylinders. Hyperbaric personnel should be familiar with these guidelines. Read the departmental emergency procedures. Keep and read the material safety data sheets on the gases used in the facility. Always check the cylinder's label before using. The cylinder and valve assembly should be inspected for damage. Valves should only be hand tight, and they should be opened slowly. The gas inside the cylinder should be compatible with the regulator. Cylinders should be secured to the wall. Keep full and empty cylinders separate, and mark the area with signs. Leak check fittings and valves with a soap-and-water solution. If a cylinder is found to be leaking, remove it from service and place in a well-ventilated storage area.

Safety guideline "dont's" to be followed for gas cylinders

For gas cylinder safety, follow these simple rules: Do not lift a cylinder by the valve cap or assembly. Always use a cylinder cart with attached chain to move cylinders. If a cylinder is deeply scratched or dented, take it out of service. Be sure the cylinder is labeled, and always read the label before use. Do not use force to open a valve or try to lubricate any part of the cylinder. If a valve cannot be opened by hand, it cannot be safely closed in an emergency. Do not mix gases or try to fill gas from one cylinder to another. Do not use the same cylinder storage area for flammable and nonflammable gases, and do not store cylinders in temperatures greater than 125° Fahrenheit. Do not touch a cylinder with your bare skin in freezing weather. Do not switch the regulators on cylinders.

Potential emergency situations that could occur during chamber operations

A hyperbaric facility is required to have protocols in place for all potential emergency situations. Common patient emergency examples are a central nervous system oxygen-toxicity seizure, a suspected pneumothorax, an unresponsive patient or cardiac arrest, and an incapacitated chamber operator. Common chamber emergencies could involve a loss of chamber pressurization, a loss of treatment gas, an uncontrollable increase in pressure, a fire inside or outside the chamber, an oxygen leak, a loss of communications, and a stuck door locking pin. Other situations that may require chamber operator assistance or attentiveness but that may not be designated as emergency situations include anxiety or escalating neuroses, labored breathing, hypoglycemia symptoms, or patient complaints. All facility emergency procedures must be followed.

<u>Emergency protocol for oxygen issues inside the chamber</u>
A suspected oxygen leak may be confirmed by the use of a mixture of soap and water (Snoop) sprayed at the leak site. If there is determined to be a leakage of oxygen coming from the chamber, try to determine the source of the leak if possible. If the technologist can correct the oxygen leak without disturbing the patient, he or she may attempt to do so. The hyperbaric physician and nurse must be notified of the situation to determine and direct patient care actions as appropriate. The usual culprit for chamber oxygen leakage is the door gasket. The gasket is the rubber barrier between the door and the chamber, which makes the gas-tight seal of the chamber possible. It is prudent to keep an extra door gasket on hand to facilitate repairs quickly and efficiently so as not to interrupt the continuity of the daily patient flow. Schedule other repairs as needed, and document actions in the chamber manual.

Emergency protocol for pressure issues inside the chamber

If a loss of chamber pressure is detected inside the hyperbaric chamber, the technologist may adjust the rate of decompression by lowering the ventilation control valve, typically located on the underside of the chamber. The patient must be notified of the treatment coming to an end. The hyperbaric physician should be notified as well. The manufacturer of the monoplace chamber has designed the chamber to self-decompress at a low rate if the chamber gas supply has been lost. The parameters of the ventilation valve are 80 to 400 liters per minute (Lpm). Adjusting the ventilation valve to 120 Lpm gives a decompression rate of 1.5 psi/minute for a typical hyperbaric chamber. Consult the user manual for chamber-specific rates. The reason for loss of chamber pressure must be determined and repairs scheduled as necessary prior to resuming treatments. An uncontrollable increase in chamber pressure may also occur. The primary action to take is to secure the gas supply and to let the chamber decompress on its own or control the decompression with the ventilation valve. Again, determine the reason and schedule repairs. All actions must be documented in the chamber manual.

Emergency protocol for loss of power and/or communication issues inside the chamber

If there is a loss of communications within the chamber, the technologist must notify the hyperbaric physician to determine if it is appropriate to continue with the treatment. If the patient is depressurizing or at depth, use flash cards to communicate with the patient and determine if it is okay to continue with the treatment. If the chamber is pressurizing, stop travel and proceed with the aforementioned steps. If the treatment needs to be aborted, ascend at a normal rate. If there is a loss of power inside the chamber, stop travel and switch to battery power. Determine the cause of the power loss and correct or repair if possible. The hyperbaric physician will determine if it is appropriate to finish the treatment. Once the chamber is switched to battery power, there will be enough power to finish a complete hyperbaric treatment. Schedule repairs as needed and document actions in chamber manual.

Emergency protocol for a patient having a seizure inside the chamber

All patients must be monitored for signs and symptoms of central nervous system oxygen toxicity: vision changes, ear ringing, nausea, tingling/twitching, irritability, dizziness, and convulsions (acronymized as VENTID-C). If possible inside the chamber, immediately place all patients showing any indication of oxygen toxicity on an air mask. Notify the physician at the first sign of a seizure. Do not ascend the chamber until verification can be made that the patient is breathing normally. Ascend the patient at a safe rate per the hyperbaric physician's instructions, which may be 3 psi/minute or slower depending on the patient's condition. Continue to watch for signs of apnea. Stop travel immediately if the seizure recurs or if the patient stops breathing. Attempt to communicate with the patient. Once the patient is on the surface, assess the airway, breathing, and vital signs including blood glucose level. Be sure to document all actions.

Emergency protocol for suspected pneumothorax inside the chamber

A pneumothorax is a collapsed lung. If the technologist suspects a pneumothorax inside the hyperbaric chamber, stop travel immediately and notify the hyperbaric physician and the nurse. Maintain a constant depth until it is determined that the treatment should be terminated. The symptoms of a pneumothorax include shortness of breath, a sudden onset of sharp chest pain that is made worse by a cough or a deep breath, nasal flaring, and fatigue. The skin may develop a bluish tint. When the hyperbaric physician determines that termination is needed, depressurize the chamber using a slow descent rate, and watch the patient carefully for signs of apnea. Make sure that the emergency response is activated. Once the patient exits the chamber, the physician should use the stethoscope to listen for decreased or absent breath sounds over the affected lung. As always, be sure to document all actions in the patient's chart.

Emergency protocol for unresponsive patient/cardiac arrest inside the chamber

It is important to be familiar with all emergency procedures concerning hyperbaric chambers. The actions taken upon recognition of an unresponsive/cardiac arrest patient are most critical for chamber operators to understand. Emergency protocols for handling unresponsive patients varies for monoplace versus multiplace chambers. For monoplace chambers, cease chamber travel in order to maintain a constant depth. Next, notify the medical director and the registered nurse on duty to immediately call a code or contact 911. Then, initiate emergency response decompression via ascending the patient to the surface at 5 psi/minute. Upon evacuation of the chamber, be sure to clear all oxygen-saturated linen before transferring the patient to a nonhyperbaric stretcher. Where applicable, assist the cardiac arrest team with cardiopulmonary resuscitation, defibrillation, or relocation of the patient to the emergency room. Within multiplace chambers, a tender may either apply standard resuscitative procedures (with precaution) or safely decompress the patient to allow the cardiac arrest team to proceed. Any emergency incidents should be documented by the chamber operator.

Emergency protocol for an incapacitated chamber operator inside or outside the chamber

If a chamber operator suddenly becomes incapacitated, the remaining medical staff should stop travel in the chamber if pressurizing and maintain depth until directed to continue or abort treatment per the hyperbaric physician. Call the code team or emergency medical services (EMS). If the physician directs the medical staff to abort the treatment, make the travel rate 2 psi/minute, and make the pressure set to the lowest setting (1.5 psi or zero). If the inside tender becomes incapacitated, notify the hyperbaric physician and call a code or EMS. Use the medical/personnel lock to lock in a member of the medical staff, or bring the whole chamber up to the surface, as directed by the hyperbaric physician. If symptoms of decompression sickness are experienced by the tender, contact the Divers Alert Network immediately.

Protocol for addressing patient complaints inside the chamber

If the patient indicates that he or she has a complaint while inside the chamber, stop travel if the chamber is changing pressure, and communicate with the patient to try and determine the nature of the complaint. Be ready to notify the hyperbaric physician and the nurse if needed. If you can easily resolve the complaint, the treatment may resume as before. If the patient complains of symptoms of oxygen toxicity, stop travel and switch the patient to an air mask if available and notify the hyperbaric physician. If the patient complains of claustrophobia, or confinement anxiety and you cannot resolve it, then safely decompress the chamber and notify the hyperbaric physician and the nurse. The patient's status should be determined after termination of the treatment. Be sure to document all actions in the patient's chart.

Protocol for a stuck door-locking pin on the chamber

If at the completion of a treatment in the hyperbaric chamber the chamber door will not open, you should check to see if the chamber door-locking pin is stuck in place. The protocol to remove the locking pin and open the chamber door is to insert a nonmetallic blunt object into the pinhole, such as a plastic pen cap or a plastic highlighter, and push the locking pin back into its seated position. Then proceed to open the chamber door. You may use an approved oxygen-safe lubricant on the door-locking pin. If the problem persists, call the chamber manufacturer for the required maintenance, and take the chamber out of service until the issue can be resolved. Document all actions in the chamber manual.

Emergency protocol for encountering a prohibited item inside of the chamber

If the hyperbaric technologist discovers a patient has a prohibited item inside a chamber, the technologist must stop travel immediately if descending. Communicate to the patient without alarming him or her that you are stopping the treatment. Ascend the chamber to the surface at a quick but controlled rate. Remove the item and the patient from the chamber. Notify the hyperbaric physician of the situation and seek direction. The patient must be reeducated about which items are permitted and which are prohibited and why. If the patient was not responsible for the prohibited item, a review of the patient predive checklist must be initiated. Always communicate any incident to the supervisor. The physician will decide whether or not to continue with the treatment. As always, document your actions.

Emergency protocol for fire inside or outside of the chamber

If a fire alarm is sounded outside of the chamber, verify that the fire is in the immediate vicinity requiring chamber evacuation as required by the facility protocol. Bring the patient up from depth at a safe rate, which may be up to 5 psi/minute as directed by the hyperbaric physician. Verify that the emergency response system has been activated. Once the chamber has surfaced, evacuate all patients by the means appropriate to the patient (stretcher, wheelchair, ambulatory). Close the chamber door and turn off the oxygen supply valve. If the fire is known to be an exercise or drill, follow the facility policy. All staff must participate in a fire exercise, all chambers must be simulated to be at deepest treatment depth, and all actions must be documented for a subsequent critique. If the fire is inside the chamber, use the emergency vent to bring the chamber up to the surface in less than 2 minutes, and follow physician instructions.

Types and components of fire suppression systems

The fire suppression system in the hyperbaric facility is governed by the National Fire Protection Association Health Care Facilities Code 99 (NFPA 99). The multiplace chamber has a water spray protection system installed. This system can handle unique environments. This water spray system's discharge is dependent on the chamber square footage. The type of water spray is deluge, and it must be independently supplied and piped. The deluge system sprays large amounts of water in a short time over the whole chamber area. The second part of the fire suppression system for the multiplace chamber is the handlines. These are manually operated fire hoses. The number of handlines depends on the chamber square footage. The deluge system is controlled on the exterior chamber console, whereas the handlines may be operated by the inside tender.

Routine maintenance necessary to ensure fire suppression system performance

The fire suppression system in the hyperbaric facility is governed by the National Fire Protection Association Health Care Facilities Code 99 (NFPA 99). During the design and installation process, the water pressure and flow requirements must be calculated accurately to provide ample water delivery. Nozzle diameter, water pressure, flow, spray pattern, and friction all contribute to the water distribution in the chamber. The spray nozzles inside the chamber must have an even distribution pattern for best extinguishing ability. Another consideration in fire suppression system design for hyperbaric chamber use is the maximum depth at which the chamber treats patients. The nozzle has to have a working pressure over chamber pressure to function. The pipes and water tanks must be made of nonferrous material. Local water source content must be analyzed before deciding the best materials for water storage. All water systems must be function tested according to a specific schedule.

Various inspection schedule increments for the fire suppression system

All water systems must be function tested according to a specific schedule. The testing procedures for properly inspecting, maintaining, and testing water extinguishing systems may be found under the NFPA regulations. Daily schedule: measure the tank and system pressure in the piping system and at the console, measure the water levels in the tanks, test all control valve positions, check visually for nozzle obstructions. Monthly schedule: complete all daily inspections, test the water flow using the by-pass valve (alternate switch actuation). Quarterly schedule: complete all daily and monthly inspections, use the opposite switch from the last monthly inspection, test the water flow with the by-pass valve. Annual schedule: complete the daily, monthly and quarterly inspections; visually inspect the piping, water tank, nozzles, controls and handlines; discharge the system completely by use of hoses attached to the piping.

Pure oxygen under pressure

Inside the monoplace hyperbaric chamber is an atmosphere containing pure (100%) oxygen. Three elements must be present for a fire to exist: heat, fuel, and an oxidizer (oxygen). In an atmosphere with normal air, a spark is harmless, but in an environment with enriched oxygen, the same harmless spark may cause a fire. In a pure-oxygen atmosphere under pressure, the spark may cause an explosion. If this explosion happens inside the hyperbaric chamber, the explosion under pressure will likely cause the chamber end caps to blow off, and possibly shatter the acrylic. Anyone in the vicinity of the chamber explosion will be in danger of losing their lives. These facts must always be in the forefront of the mind of the hyperbaric technologist as he or she goes about completing items on the daily chamber checklist and the patient checklist.

Items permitted inside of a chamber

Items that are approved to be inside a hyperbaric chamber include: plastic urinals, emesis basins, certain types of drains, intravenous (IV) lines without a green or orange cap (the caps contain alcohol solution), catheters, nasogastric tubes, stoma bags, tampons or sanitary napkins, and water bottles without the label as long as the patient is educated on leaving the cap loose in the pressurized chamber. Blankets, sheets, pillowcases, and gowns may go inside the chamber if they are either 100% cotton, or a 50% cotton/polyester blend. Total-contact casts and nail polish are approved as long as they have been cured for at least 10 hours. Pacemakers, defibrillators, and medication pumps are allowed with the manufacturer's approval in writing. Certain topical wound care medications, the electrodes and fixation rings of a $tcPO_2$ monitor, nonrebreather masks for air breaks, and special IV pumps adapted for pressure are also allowed.

Materials and substances not permitted inside of a chamber

The hyperbaric chamber contains 100% oxygen at a higher than normal pressure, and under certain conditions, there is a great risk of fire. There must be three things for a fire to exist: oxygen, heat, and fuel. The oxygen factor cannot be removed, but heat and fuel can be limited by prohibiting potentially flammable items inside of the chamber. The list of prohibited materials and substances include but are not limited to street clothes and shoes, linens that are not at least 51% cotton, oil-/petroleum-based skin and hair products, wigs or hairpieces, heating/cooling patches, cigarettes, matches, and lighters. If the patient was not born with it, it does not belong in the chamber. Taking appropriate measures to educate patients on risks as well as thoroughly checking for contraband prior to pressurization will greatly reduce the possibility of a chamber fire.

Electronic devices not permitted inside of a chamber

The hyperbaric chamber contains 100% oxygen at a higher than normal pressure, and under certain conditions, there is a great risk of fire. Battery-operated and electronic devices are banned, including watches, heating blankets, toys, hearing aids, cellular phones, electronic readers, and tablets. If the patient was not born with it, it does not belong in the chamber. To prevent any static electricity, the patient must be grounded to the chamber by the grounding bracelet and cord. Taking appropriate measures to educate patients on risks as well as thoroughly checking for contraband prior to pressurization will greatly reduce the possibility of a chamber fire.

Risks associated with bringing contraband into the chamber

It is very important that the patient be educated on exactly what items are prohibited inside a hyperbaric chamber. Unapproved items are prohibited for a reason. The patient's safety is the top priority of the hyperbaric technologist. Fire is the greatest risk inside the pressurized chamber with 100% oxygen. The items that are not allowed inside the chamber either cause a fire or contribute to a fire. Electronic devices, such as cell phones, may exhibit a tiny spark into the oxygen, possibly igniting a fire. If a prohibited item is discovered with a patient inside a chamber, bring the chamber to the surface immediately and reeducate the patient on the importance of keeping those items out of the chamber. With the physician's approval, the technologist may repressurize the chamber and complete the treatment.

Monoplace chamber vs. multiplace chamber

Monoplace hyperbaric chamber operation includes the following steps: Inspect chamber. Turn on the oxygen. Switch on the master valve control. Adjust the rate set of chamber travel. Adjust the pressure set to the depth the chamber is traveling to. Ensure that the air is connected and tested for possible air breaks. When the treatment is over, adjust the rate set and pressure set to idle depth, and turn off the master valve. The chamber must be completely depressurized before opening the chamber door. Multiplace chamber operation includes the following steps: Check or turn on the compressor, fire suppression system, hoods/masks, and the chamber. Turn on the air and oxygen. Ensure that the patient's hoods or masks have tight seals. Turn on the master valve. Set the rate and the pressure to the required depth. Monitor the gas analyzers and the gas selection. When the treatment is over, adjust the rate set and pressure set to idle depth and turn off the master valve. Patient preparation is the same for both chamber types.

Characteristics
A monoplace (class B) hyperbaric chamber is an enclosed acrylic tube that houses one human occupant only. A multiplace (class A) hyperbaric chamber is a room that can be pressurized and houses multiple human occupants. A monoplace chamber does not have a fire suppression system, but only an emergency vent button in case of a fire inside the chamber. A multiplace chamber has a very complex fire suppression system for chamber fires. The monoplace chamber is filled and pressurized with 100% oxygen, and it is constantly vented. The patients may take air breaks from disposable nonrebreather masks inside the chamber. The multiplace chamber is pressurized with air, and it must use oxygen, carbon dioxide, carbon monoxide, and nitrogen analyzers to determine air quality. These chamber occupants breathe 100% oxygen from masks or hoods.

Regulatory agencies related to hyperbaric oxygen therapy

The National Board of Diving and Hyperbaric Medical Technology (NBDHMT) certifies hyperbaric technologists. The National Fire Protection Association (NFPA) provides fire safety regulations. The American Society of Mechanical Engineers (ASME) provides general safety standards and codes. The ASME standard of pressure vessels for human occupancy (PVHO-1 and PCHO-2) gives regulations for chamber pressurization and acrylic. The Undersea and Hyperbaric Medicine Society (UHMS) provides accreditation standards. These regulatory agencies work together and complement each other as they strive toward best practices for hyperbaric medicine and operations.

Scope of pressure vessels for human occupancy (PVHO-1)

A PVHO-1 is any vessel or chamber under pressure that encloses a human being. Manufacturers of pressure vessels or chambers are required to hold a valid certificate of authorization for use provided by the American Society of Mechanical Engineers. The scope of this organization gives the regulations and safety standards for pressure vessels exceeding 2 psi with regard to their design, fabrication, inspection, testing, and marking. "PVHO-1" is to be stamped on the pressure vessel or chamber when it has met these requirements. Piping systems for pressure vessels also fall under these regulations with regard to their design, fabrication, inspection, testing, cleaning, and certification. This applies to repairs made at current facilities and new construction as well. Some of the vessels that fall under this standard are submersibles, diving bells, personnel transfer capsules, decompression chambers, recompression chambers, hyperbaric chambers, high-altitude chambers, and medical hyperbaric oxygenation facilities.

Scope of pressure vessels for human occupancy (PVHO-2)

PVHO-2 is a pressure vessel for human occupancy. The American Society of Mechanical Engineers gives regulations and safety standards for acrylic windows with regard to their in-service inspection, care, repair, replacement, testing, and recertification. The responsibility for determining the safe service life with regard to the technical criteria and guidelines is not of the designer or fabricator, but of the user of the pressure vessel in which the acrylic is housed, and he or she can determine when the acrylic requires replacement. The acrylic windows that are in service should be visually inspected before use each day. If the chamber is pressurized multiple times a day, one inspection on the first pressurization will suffice. The inspection includes checking for the presence of crazing, discoloration, cracks, chips, scratches, gouges, burns, and pits that could affect the structural integrity of the acrylic window.

Clinical Skills (supervised)

NFPA 99, chapter 14

The National Fire Protection Association Health Care Facilities Code 99 (NFPA 99) is the standard for healthcare facilities. Chapter 14 deals with hyperbaric facilities. NFPA regulations for hyperbaric facilities consist of chamber classifications, construction and equipment, housing for hyperbaric facilities, chamber fabrication, illumination, chamber ventilation, sources of air for multiplace chamber atmospheres, temperature and humidity control, fire protection, emergency procedures, deluge systems, handline systems, fire detection, testing, electrical systems, personnel, and gas systems. The NFPA also gives instruction on textiles (garments worn in hyperbaric chambers), flammable gases and liquids, ignition sources, safeguards, and maintenance.

Different biomedical devices used within the hyperbaric facility

The patient's vital signs are taken before and after every hyperbaric treatment. These may be taken manually by the hyperbaric technologist or nurse, but sometimes a biomedical device called a blood pressure or vitals machine is used. This may be a Welch Allyn machine, or it may be from another vendor. It can be used to record blood pressure, pulse, temperature, and oxygen saturation and has the ability to print out results. Another device used in the facility is the blood glucometer for diabetic patients. Before use, this meter must be tested every day with quality control liquids. The patient lift, or Hoyer lift, is a device used to pick up a patient and transfer him or her from one chair or bed to another chair or bed. This is achieved by use of a canvas sling and a mechanical lift.

Properly conducting an assessment of the patient for pain

Many hyperbaric patients may have pain during the course of their treatments. The technologist must assess the pain and communicate with the hyperbaric nurse and/or physician to determine the correct course of action. A pain assessment is conducted by asking the patient to rate their pain on a scale of 1 to 10, with 1 being slight discomfort and 10 being the worst pain ever. Some facilities may have a chart posted to help the patient determine their pain level. This chart is usually made up of faces depicted in a cartoonish manner along a scale from 1 to 10. Each face is a little more distressed than the last, until the final face shows excruciating pain. If the patient is in too much pain to go through with their hyperbaric treatment, the physician may prescribe a pain medication. If the patient states a point of relief after a certain period of time, the technologist may proceed with the chamber treatment.

Importance of obtaining vital signs

It is important that the patient's vital signs be taken before and after every hyperbaric treatment. The vital signs consist of the blood glucose level (BGL), blood pressure, pulse, respirations, temperature, and oxygen saturation level. The BGL of a diabetic patient must be about 110 to 130 mg/dl to qualify for a chamber treatment because a mechanism in the body reacts to the chamber pressure by dropping the BGL about 50 mg/dl. The BGL must be checked after the treatment to make sure the patient is stable. The blood pressure may be checked with a vitals machine, or it may be checked manually. A manual blood pressure check tends to be more accurate. The pulse, temperature, and O_2 saturation may also be checked using the vitals machine. It is important to take vital signs after a hyperbaric treatment because the vitals may be the only way to determine if the patient has had a negative reaction inside the chamber.

Qualifying for a hyperbaric chamber treatment

Parameters for the pulse of a patient

In order to qualify for a hyperbaric treatment, the patient's pulse must not show bradycardia, which is less than 60 bpm (beats per minute), nor must the patient have tachycardia, which is more than 100 bpm. If the patient has either of these symptoms, the hyperbaric physician must be notified. These symptoms do not necessarily mean a dive cancellation. The physician may decide to intervene with medications or other treatment prior to the dive. If there is an irregular heart rate noted predive or postdive, the physician must be notified. Bradycardia or tachycardia may indicate that a new or existing cardiac problem has arisen. The patient's other vital signs should be taken, for a full picture of the issue. At this point, the physician will make the decision on whether or not to proceed with the patient's treatment.

Parameters for patient's blood pressure

In order to qualify for a hyperbaric chamber treatment, the patient's blood pressure must be within certain parameters. The patient's systolic blood pressure must be no less than 100 mmHg and no greater than 180 mmHg. The patient's diastolic blood pressure must be no less than 60 mmHg and no greater than 100 mmHg. For any occurrence outside of these parameters, the hyperbaric physician must be notified. If a patient has just come from dialysis and has a low blood pressure, he or she may only need to be hydrated. Reference the patient's chart and coordinate with the hyperbaric nurse on this issue. If the patient's blood pressure is too high, the physician might order medication prior to hyperbaric treatment. A 15- to 30-minute wait is usually required before retaking the blood pressure.

Parameters for patient's temperature

In order to qualify for a hyperbaric treatment the patient's temperature must meet certain parameters. The patient's temperature must be taken before hyperbaric treatment is started. The oral temperature must be no greater than 101° Fahrenheit. If the patient's temperature is above 101°, the hyperbaric physician must be notified. The physician may treat the patient with an antipyretic prior to hyperbaric treatment. The patient must not undergo a hyperbaric treatment with a high temperature because it would cause the patient to be more susceptible to an oxygen-toxicity seizure. After the medication is administered, wait 15 to 30 minutes before rechecking the temperature. If the patient is stable, proceed with the dive under physician supervision.

Parameters for patient's respiration rate

The respiration rate for adults is typically 12 to 24 breaths per minute. Before a treatment in a hyperbaric chamber, record the patient's respiration rate. If the patient is noted to have labored breathing or an abnormal respiration rate, notify the physician immediately. These symptoms may be caused by a more serious medical problem. If spontaneous abnormal breathing occurs in the hyperbaric chamber, notify the hyperbaric physician immediately. The dive may need to be aborted or shortened, depending on the patient's status. If the dive needs to be aborted, be sure to watch the patient closely for signs of apnea. If the patient stops breathing, stop travel and consult the physician.

Parameters for patient's blood sugar

The blood glucose level (BGL) of a diabetic patient must be taken before and after a hyperbaric treatment. The parameters for the BGL are 110–130 mg/dl to 250–300 mg/dl, depending on the physician's discretion and the facility policy. If the patients BGL is too low, hypoglycemic interventions may be taken, such as giving the patient an Ensure or Glucerna or equivalent product. Crackers and peanut butter may also be given. Wait 30 minutes to retest the BGL. Be sure to ask the patient when he or she last ate a meal and when their last dose of insulin was taken. This may impact the BGL readings. If the BGL is too high, insulin may be given at the physician's discretion, but it may also be prudent to cancel the dive for that day.

Parameters for patient's oxygen saturation

If the patient's oxygen saturation reading is below 94%, he or she may not be stable enough to undergo a hyperbaric treatment. Although the 100% oxygen may be good for the patient, being in an enclosed space that is not readily accessible to medical staff may be risky. Ultimately, it is at the physician's discretion whether or not to have the patient undergo the hyperbaric oxygen therapy for the day. If the patient comes into the hyperbaric suite on an oxygen nasal cannula or nonrebreather mask, be sure to take that into account when measuring the patient's oxygen saturation. If possible, take the patient off of the oxygen for 10 minutes before measuring the oxygen saturation.

Signs and symptoms observed when there is a change is neurological status

Neurological changes in patients can happen quickly during hyperbaric oxygen treatments. The hyperbaric technologist should be familiar with the signs and symptoms that may foretell a neurological status change. Getting to know the patient's personality and mannerisms at the beginning of the treatment program is essential to understanding what signifies normal or abnormal behavior for the patient. This makes it easier to notice when there is an extreme behavioral modification such as illogical/uncontrollable, emotional, or physical reactions. Sudden irritability is a common symptom for neurological changes such as a hypoglycemic episode or a prelude to an oxygen-toxicity seizure. Excessive sweating, shaking/shivering, hand or face twitching, and slurring of speech are all signs and symptoms to look for when evaluating neurological status.

Applying the sterile technique

During hyperbaric operations and ancillary services, it is sometimes imperative to keep a sterile field. During wound care and assisting in debridement especially, the technologist must develop a sterile technique. The tools, instruments, wound care products, and equipment used when dealing with open wounds must not only be cleaned but also be sterilized. Products such as gauze and tools such as cleaned scissors have the potential for the onloading of bacteria, which could lead to infection in the patient. To create a sterile field, gather all the items needed in one place. Wash your hands properly, glove up, and wear a mask and a gown. Use double-wrapped packaging for all sterile equipment and unwrap from the edges without passing your hands over the sterile field. Repeat this process for all items.

Collecting and removung medical waste products

In a hyperbaric and wound care facility, medical waste products may accumulate from time to time. This waste must be collected and removed in a particular way. Examples of medical waste would be blood, body-fluid-stained gauze or wound dressings, needles, emesis, feces, and urine to name a few. The collection process must be done with the appropriate protective gear. Gowns, gloves, protective foot wear, masks, and face shields are examples of body substance isolation gear available to the technologist. The medical waste product must be disposed of in a biohazard bag or box, or a sharps container as appropriate. The patients who require hyperbaric treatments are generally very sick, and they may have infectious diseases. Because it may not be known if a particular patient suffers from an infectious disease, it is imperative that all medical waste products be treated as potential biohazards.

Maintaining privacy when working with multiple patients in a hyperbaric facility

The hyperbaric suite may have multiple monoplace chambers, or it may have a multiplace chamber. If that is the case, an effort must be made to maintain patient privacy when multiple patients are being treated hyperbarically. Calling out personal information in front of other patients is not wise or allowed by law (the Health Insurance Portability and Accountability Act). Most facilities are equipped with curtains that may be pulled for patient privacy. Even if the patient does not voice a desire not to be seen by other patients, the technologist should assume that all patients desire their privacy whether they are bedbound and changing their gown or if their wounds are being assessed. Being in a hurry to fill the chambers does not trump the need for patient privacy. This may slow the process down, but it may also give the technologist a good opportunity to ensure that the patient has no contraband on their person prior to their chamber treatment.

Assisting in wound dressing changes

From time to time, the hyperbaric technologist may be called upon to perform wound dressing changes for patients undergoing hyperbaric therapy. The technologist must be checked off on every procedure by a nurse before performing such duties. Furthermore, wound dressing changes may not take place inside the hyperbaric suite, nor may the changes take place inside a hyperbaric chamber. The patient must be taken into an exam room to be assessed and to have wound dressing changes completed. This is in accordance with NFPA 99. The hyperbaric technologist may do any wound care or dressing changes under the supervision of a registered nurse and may receive training and certification for such, as long as he or she is signed off by the nurse.

Assisting in otologic procedures

During the course of hyperbaric chamber treatments, a patient may have problems equalizing the ears, or have pain in the ears. When this occurs, the nurse and hyperbaric physician must be notified so as to decide the course of action. The physician may decide the patient needs to have pressure equalization (PE) tubes inserted into the eardrums, or he or she may decide that the patient's ears need to be irrigated. If the patient requires PE tubes before further hyperbaric treatments, the technologist may make an appointment for the patient with an ear, nose, and throat doctor. If the patient requires irrigation, this procedure may be done in an exam room if the physician is comfortable with the procedure.

The technologist should periodically inspect the patient's ears with an otoscope depending on the Teed (after Wallace Teed, a U.S. submariner during World War II) scale for clarification. The Teed scale should be posted in the hyperbaric suite.

Assisting in an electrocardiogram test

The potential hyperbaric patient may be required by the physician to have completed an electrocardiogram (EKG or ECG) prior to undergoing hyperbaric treatment. Depending on your facility policy, the technologist may make the patient an appointment with a cardiologist, or, in a hospital facility, the technologist may call for an EKG to be performed in the exam room. If the technologist is certified, he or she may perform the EKG. The patient may be having cardiac issues during the hyperbaric treatment, if this is the case, the physician may order an EKG to be done immediately. The technologist must either perform the EKG or call an EKG stat code to the department. The patient must be reevaluated before resuming or restarting hyperbaric treatments.

Quality control steps taken to ensure compliance for a glucometer

Every day, the glucometer for blood glucose tests must be quality control tested before it is used for patient blood glucose testing. There are two types of glucometer control liquids: a high control, and a low control. These controls are typically supplied by the hospital's laboratory department. The low control is typically done first. First, turn on the glucometer and provide your personal ID code. Then select "quality control." The meter will take you through the steps. Scan or enter the glucose strip lot number. Scan or enter the low-control lot number. Insert a glucose strip into the glucometer. When the screen indicates ready, squeeze one drop of the low-control liquid onto the strip. After a few seconds, the screen will read either PASS or FAIL. Follow the on-screen directions for either result. Repeat the same steps for the high control. Every glucometer is different, but these steps are generally the same.

Standard hyperbaric education provided to new patients

The patient must be assessed by the hyperbaric physician and the nurse prior to receiving hyperbaric education from the technologist. The patient should be made to feel as comfortable as possible when considering hyperbaric treatment. If possible, physically show the patients the hyperbaric suite and the chambers. Explain how the chambers pressurize and depressurize, and explain how the patient should equalize his or her own ears (have them demonstrate) during the treatments. Educate the patient on approved and prohibited items inside the chamber. The patient must know what skin and hair products may or may not be used prior to chamber treatments. The patient must also be made aware of the dangers of bringing any electronic devices into the hyperbaric chamber. The patient must know the signs and symptoms of oxygen toxicity. They must be told to breathe normally at all times inside the chamber and also that their vision may change during the course of their treatments. The technologist must explain the comforts and entertainments that may be had inside the chamber and how important it is to be consistent with the treatment schedule.

Positioning your body and the patient's body for transfers and off-loading

When transferring a patient, every effort must be made to keep the patient as comfortable as possible, but above all, the technologist must not put him or herself in a position to become hurt or injured during a transfer. Education on body positional transfers must be given to the technologist upon request. When in doubt during a patient transfer, always ask for help. Transfer equipment, such as slide boards and lifts must be available to the technologist. For a one-man transfer from a wheelchair to a bed, position the wheelchair at a 45-degree angle to the bed after asking the patient which side he or she prefers to transfer from. Lock the wheels and detach or move the wheelchair legs. Position your knees in front of the patient's knees, and instruct the patient to lift from the armrests using the arms. Hold the patient either under the armpits or by the gait belt. When the patient is standing, have him or her make small steps to turn the backside toward the bed, and then lower the patient onto the bed. Grab the patient by the upper back and under the knees, and then pivot on the patient's backside until the body is in line with the bed. Lay the patient down. Be sure to offload the patient's heel with a blanket or a towel to prevent pressure sores.

Garments that should or should not be worn inside of the chamber

Garments worn by patients or inside tenders inside a hyperbaric chamber should be made of either 100% cotton, or of a 50% cotton/polyester blend. The patient should be educated on the type of clothing allowed inside the monoplace chamber. Most hyperbaric facilities have either patient gowns and pants or scrubs tops and bottoms that are made of approved materials. Patients must be made aware that he or she may not use underwear not provided by the facility. Socks may be available upon request as well. The patient may not bring anything into the chamber except his or her body. The rules are slightly different with multiplace chambers. The atmosphere in a multiplace chamber is not 100% oxygen, so the patient may have items such as socks and underwear. The patient may also be allowed to have items such as books and magazines. Facility policy must dictate any special circumstances.

Orientation process for elderly patients

The hyperbaric oxygen therapy education process for elderly patients must be handled with finesse. These are typically very sick patients who are on their last-ditch effort to heal. If the family is present, it is usually best to involve them if possible. The technologist's discretion is needed here because sometimes the family may be apathetic toward the patient and/or the treatment. If that is the case, direct the education toward the patient only and let him or her know that you have their best interests in mind. You are the patient's advocate. The orientation to the chamber and the commitment to treatment must be presented in such a way that the patient can see themselves being successful for the duration of the treatments. The patient should be shown the chamber, the gurney, where they would be changing clothes, and where their personal belongings would be secured, and patients should be introduced to all staff. It is the responsibility of all staff to be a part of the education process and to make the patient feel comfortable by practicing empathy and patience.

Orientation process for pediatric patients

The hyperbaric technologist must be as kind and gentle as possible when attempting to educate a pediatric patient about hyperbaric oxygen therapy. Most likely, the pediatric patient will be nervous about the reason for the treatment in the first place, and then to be told he or she has to be inside of a scary chamber is even worse. The technologist should not talk down to the patient, but describe the process as simply as possible as if speaking with an adult. The technologist should describe the entire hyperbaric treatment process as if telling a story. The patient's family will most likely be encouraging to the process, so it is best to involve them in the story as much as possible. The patient and the family should be given a tour of the hyperbaric suite and shown how a chamber works. The technologist should be aware that he or she is educating the family as much as the patient. Having a compassionate yet confident bedside manner makes a big difference.

Best ways to address patient discomfort

Patient discomfort inside the hyperbaric chamber should be addressed on a case-by-case basis. The patient should feel that they are able to communicate with the technologist freely, and that they are in sight at all times during the hyperbaric treatment. The best way to treat patient discomfort inside the chamber is to prevent it in the first place. Be sure to provide enough blankets and pillows, and position patients so that they are physically comfortable before starting the treatment. Limit the amount of noises in the hyperbaric suite that may startle the patient. Do not lean on or bump the chamber during the treatment. After all preventive measures have been taken; the patient may still express discomfort inside the chamber. Listen carefully to the patient's concerns and address them with compassion. If needed, call the hyperbaric physician or nurse to come over and provide extra reassurance to the patient. Patients should understand they have control and are able to request for the treatment to be ceased.

Generalized Clinical Knowledge

Risks, side effects, and dangers associated with various drugs

Aspirin

Aspirin is a mild pain reliever that is nonnarcotic. This and other nonsteroidal anti-inflammatory drugs such as acetaminophen and Motrin, when taken in the correct dosage specifications, have not shown any negative effects when used in conjunction with hyperbaric oxygen therapy (HBOT) as related to oxygen toxicity. The effects of these medications under the influence of oxygen partial pressures do not seem to be impaired. Some schools of thought believe that aspirin may give the potential for oxygen toxicity, but this has never been proved, nor has there been any evidence to substantiate these claims. Aspirin and other nonnarcotic medications are not contraindicated for HBOT.

Cis-platinum

Cis-platinum is a chemotherapeutic drug that is used in certain cancers such as head, neck, testicular, and ovarian cancers. This drug works against DNA synthesis; therefore, it affects the production of fibroblasts and the synthesis of collagen. This process impedes wound healing. During animal testing for this drug, HBOT was found to have an adverse effect when used concurrently with cis-platinum by increasing the cytotoxic effect in the tissues. This incompatible drug effect should not, however, be taken into account when dealing with life-threatening emergencies such carbon monoxide poisoning, necrotizing fasciitis, or gas gangrene. In these cases, the risk of cis-platinum does not outweigh the benefit of HBOT.

Doxorubicin

Adriamycin, or doxorubicin, is a drug used for a wide variety of cancers. This drug works as a type of antibiotic that affects DNA. One of its most serious side effects is damage to the heart. During animal testing for this drug, 87% of the animals were found to expire when exposed to hyperbaric oxygen (HBO) conditions. The same effect was found when HBO was implemented once a day, or twice a day when used concurrently with Adriamycin. Adriamycin (doxorubicin) is an absolute contraindication to hyperbaric oxygen therapy (HBOT), and the two should never be combined. If a patient taking Adriamycin is in need of HBOT, the drug should be stopped for at least three days before starting HBOT.

Mafenide acetate

Mafenide acetate, or Sulfamylon, is a topical cream used mostly for second- and third-degree burns. Its antibacterial properties suppress bacterial growth on burn victims. The use of mafenide acetate cream can cause a buildup of carbon dioxide, which leads to vasodilation. Hyperbaric oxygen therapy (HBOT) introduces a mechanism that causes vasoconstriction. The vasodilation of mafenide acetate and the vasoconstriction of HBOT cause a negative effect when used concurrently. If the burn patient has a need for HBOT, the mafenide acetate must be removed by showering with soap and water before treatment in a hyperbaric chamber. An alternative drug for burn patients is Silvadene cream, which is approved for HBOT.

Bleomycin

Bleomycin is an antibiotic agent used for certain types of cancers. It has been indicated in the past to be an absolute contraindication because the effects of oxygen on the patient were thought to cause bleomycin lung. Bleomycin lung typically occurs in patients at the time of their first treatment, and at only 4%. There is no evidence to prove that a patient may have a recurrence of bleomycin lung with the introduction of oxygen into the body. For precautionary measures, the hyperbaric physician may decide to do a pulmonary function test on patients with prior use of bleomycin. Although precautions with lung functioning should be taken, bleomycin is no longer contraindicated for hyperbaric oxygen therapy.

Steroids

Oxygen toxicity remains a factor when steroids are used concurrently with hyperbaric oxygen therapy (HBOT). When epinephrine and other hormones are increased, the response is a natural protective mechanism to stress. When used in conjunction with HBOT, steroids and adrenaline seem to make the patient sensitive to oxygen toxicity. In this case, the patient should be watched carefully for signs of oxygen toxicity and, if necessary, be given an anticonvulsant drug when indicated. The patient should be taking frequent air breaks during the course of hyperbaric chamber treatments. The use of steroids during HBOT is a relative contraindication.

Alcohol and smoking

Patients who consume alcohol and/or smoke during the course of their hyperbaric oxygen treatments may not receive the full benefits of HBO therapy. Patients who smoke before or after a hyperbaric treatment will reverse the effects of the treatment. Divers who drink alcohol excessively are predisposed to decompression sickness (DCS), but DCS is not a factor for the hyperbaric oxygen patient because they are immersed in 100% oxygen. Alcohol inebriation has not been shown to predispose a patient to oxygen toxicity, nor is the patient more prone to seizure activity. There is no evidence to suggest a sobering effect on an inebriated individual with a hyperbaric oxygen treatment. Patients should be educated on the risks associated with substance abuse.

Narcotics

Hyperbaric oxygen therapy can produce a slightly negative effect when used concurrently with narcotics. Patients who are taking narcotics may have an altered mental status during treatment, or the narcotic effect may run out during treatment. The patient must be watched closely for signs of lethargy and pain. More importantly, the use of narcotics may increase the risk for oxygen toxicity during hyperbaric oxygen treatments. Narcotics, such as morphine or meperidine (Demerol), may cause a decrease in respirations by reducing carbon dioxide sensitivity to the brain. This will cause a rise in the partial pressure of carbon dioxide in the tissues, which causes a dilation of brain tissue. This dilation prompts greater blood flow leading to more oxygen dissolved in the brain tissues and, therefore, a higher risk of oxygen convulsions.

Disulfiram

Disulfiram is a drug that helps patients overcome alcohol abuse by producing negative side effects when taken with alcohol. In animal studies, disulfiram (Antabuse) was tested in hyperbaric oxygen conditions. This drug, when tested on mice taken to 6 atmospheres absolute (ATA) for one hour, did not allow the mice to have oxygen-toxicity convulsions. The same result was reported when the drug was tested on dogs at 4 ATA. This test has not been repeated with human trials, but based on the animal test data, disulfiram is no longer considered a contraindication to hyperbaric oxygen therapy. Disulfiram, however, is not an approved method for preventing oxygen toxicity.

Lorazepam

Lorazepam (Ativan) is not a contraindication to hyperbaric oxygen therapy (HBOT). In fact, when used in conjunction with HBOT, Lorazepam will relieve anxiety of patients who have claustrophobia. This drug is very effective in sedating patients, and it also produces lack of recall within 15 to 20 minutes of intravenous injection. The effects of this drug can last up to eight hours. Lorazepam has been shown to be effective in the management of epilepsy, but it is not approved for that indication. Lorazepam does not affect the respiratory depressant side effect of narcotics. This drug can be a useful tool in helping patients to complete their HBOT course.

Fundamentals of practicing cardiopulmonary resuscitation

Knowledge of cardiopulmonary resuscitation (CPR) is essential to the hyperbaric technologist. It is important to be able to recognize when a patient is in distress and requires CPR. When a patient stops breathing and has no pulse, the technologist should call for help and initiate CPR immediately starting with chest compressions. Starting with 30 compressions followed by two breaths equals one cycle. Five cycles, or two minutes, of CPR must be completed before activating the automatic external defibrillator (AED). If the AED is present during a witnessed cardiac arrest, activate the AED before initiating CPR. If performing two-person CPR, be sure to switch responders between breaths and compressions often to prevent fatigue, and therefore, ineffective CPR.

Fundamentals of establishing an airway

If a patient is not breathing inside the chamber, stop travel and notify the hyperbaric physician and nurse immediately. Only depressurize the chamber when the hyperbaric physician deems it to be appropriate. Activate the emergency response system. When the chamber is on the surface, take the patient out of the chamber and transfer the patient to a nonhyperbaric hospital stretcher. Watch for chest rise and listen for breath sounds: If these are absent, open the airway by a head tilt and chin lift. If a pulse is present, attempt to give two rescue breaths. If unsuccessful, open the mouth and look for a foreign body. If located, do a finger sweep or suction. Airway adjuncts (oral or nasal) may be used on the apneic patient in order to open the airway for rescue breaths with a bag-valve mask.

Methods for managing hyperthermia

Hyperthermia is a serious condition by itself. Hyperthermia is the raising of the body temperature to above-normal levels. Normal body temperature is 98.6° Fahrenheit. If the body gets too hot, or if the patient has a temperature of greater than 104°, this is a life-threatening condition. The patient's temperature must be taken before the start of a hyperbaric treatment. If the patient's temperature is at 101° or greater, the patient must be given medication by the hyperbaric physician and the hyperbaric treatment must be delayed because at higher body temperatures, the patient is more susceptible to oxygen-toxicity seizures when inside the hyperbaric chamber.

Methods for managing hypothermia

Hypothermia is a serious medical condition in which the body's temperature drops to below normal levels. In hypothermic conditions, the body loses heat faster than it can produce heat. Hypothermia is defined as a temperature of 95° Fahrenheit or lower. Mild hypothermia is marked by shivering and confusion. Moderate hypothermia is marked by the ceasing of shivering and increased confusion. Moderate hypothermia is believed to prevent oxygen toxicity seizures in patients undergoing hyperbaric oxygen therapy because of the suppression of shivering. This method of treatment, however, is not approved, nor is it clinically practical.

Effects of 100% oxygen have on the body

High doses of oxygen under pressure can have negative side effects on the human body. The hyperbaric chamber is filled with 100% oxygen at two atmospheres absolute, two-and-a-half atmospheres absolute, and three atmospheres absolute in a clinical setting. When oxygen starts to have negative effects, it is called oxygen toxicity. There are two types of oxygen toxicity: (1) central nervous system (CNS) oxygen toxicity, which can act quickly, and (2) pulmonary oxygen toxicity, which acts slowly. The type that is most concerning for the clinical setting is CNS oxygen toxicity because there is a high risk of seizure. Several symptoms can occur before the onset of a seizure. Hyperbaric technologists use the acronym VENTID-C to identify oxygen toxicity, which represents the following: vision changes, ear ringing, nausea, tingling/twitching, irritability, and dizziness. Convulsions, representing the last letter of the acronym, are typically the only visible sign. Therefore, it is critical to encourage patients to communicate any physical or mental changes that they experience while undergoing treatment.

Effect air at pressure has on the body

When a patient or an inside tender is pressurized in a hyperbaric chamber with air, the air spaces (the middle ear, lungs, gastrointestinal tract) in the body will shrink, according to Boyle's law. The patient will be breathing 100% oxygen from a hood, but the inside tender may be breathing the air from the atmosphere. This will cause an onloading of nitrogen in the body's tissues that will need to be off-gassed appropriately, or it could cause decompression sickness. The inside tender should breathe 100% oxygen from a mask (not strapped to the head, to prevent oxygen toxicity) on a gas breathing schedule. A dive profile should be completed for any person inside the chamber that is not constantly breathing 100% oxygen from a hood.

<u>How pressure positively impacts the body</u>

A pressurized environment (hyperbaric chamber) impacts the human body in positive ways. According to Boyle's law, a pressurized environment will reduce the size of gas bubbles, such as nitrogen, in solution and in tissue. This is a positive outcome for a patient with decompression sickness. According to Henry's law, a pressurized environment will increase the amount of oxygen that is transported, dissolved in plasma, and available to tissues. The body is positively affected when breathing 100% oxygen under pressure because the hemoglobin will become overly saturated with oxygen, and at that point the plasma starts to onload oxygen as well and carry it out to the cells throughout the body. Lastly, the human body is affected positively when, by simple pressure physics, the distance at which dissolved oxygen can diffuse in tissues is increased.

Principles of decompression theory

Decompression theory accounts for the transportation of nitrogen to and from the tissues, the storage of nitrogen by the tissues, and the formation and growth of bubbles. Nitrogen transportation depends on perfusion, which is the amount of blood flow to each type of tissue; and diffusion, which is how fast nitrogen moves from the blood to the tissues, and from one tissue type to another. The capacity of a tissue to store nitrogen depends on diffusion and solubility. Solubility is the amount of gas dissolved in each tissue depending on the partial pressure of gas, type of tissue, and temperature. Bubble formation and growth are affected by the saturation of tissues: the maximum amount of gas that a tissue can uptake. Supersaturation occurs when gas tension exceeds the ambient pressure. The tissue types handle supersaturation differently. Once a bubble forms, Boyle's law comes into consideration.

Methods of ear equalization during decompression

During hyperbaric oxygen therapy (HBOT), a patient undergoes pressure changes that may lead to barotraumas if not prevented. The most common barotraumas occur in the middle-ear space. Educating a patient on how to "clear the ears" is a vital part of the HBOT orientation process. There are different methods to equalize the pressure in the middle ear. For the Valsalva maneuver, the patient is taught to pinch the nostrils, close the mouth, tighten the abdominal muscles, and blow through the nose. The Toynbee maneuver includes pinching the nostrils and swallowing. The Frenzel maneuver is closing the nostrils and throat as if straining to lift a weight, then making the letter "K" sound, which forces the back of the tongue upward, compressing air against the openings of the eustachian tubes. The Lowry technique is a combination of the Valsalva and the Toynbee: closing the nostrils, blowing, and swallowing at the same time. Other methods are simply swallowing and yawning or popping the jaw. The HBO patient can be instructed to try various methods and discover which works best.

Types of injuries that can result from improper body positioning

Body position should be the first consideration of the technologist when attempting to move a patient because it concerns safety. Not only is there a potential for injuring the patient, but there is an even bigger potential of the technologist injuring his or her own body. One mistake that a lot of technologists make is letting the patient hold onto them. This can cause an improper lift, while also keeping the patient from helping to lift their own weight. The technologist must take the time needed to position the body correctly, and to educate the patient on lift techniques. If an improper lift occurs, the pain will mostly likely not occur right away, but after a few hours or even the next day; discomfort may not resolve without medical attention. Pain may occur in the lower back, the upper back, or the neck. Some injuries require surgery, whereas others require physical therapy and pain medication.

Proper communication among all levels of the hyperbaric medical team

When the hyperbaric team communicates efficiently, the center will run smoothly. Effective and efficient communication starts with the administration and the front-desk personnel. The administration dictates by leadership and by example how the entire center will operate. When a patient makes his or her first visit to the center, the front-desk personnel have an opportunity not only to show the patient how courteously and compassionately they can expect to be treated throughout their experience, but also to gather pertinent information about the patient and how the rest of the team should plan their approach to patient care. Effective planning and communication among team members concerning wound care visits, hyperbaric treatments, and patient transportation can be achieved through team cohesion.

Practical considerations of pediatric hyperbaric treatments

Pediatric patient may benefit from hyperbaric oxygen therapy more so than their adult counterparts in the area of cellular proliferation. These younger patients may require fewer treatments for the same result. This is true for nonhealing wounds as well as radiation injuries. The maturation factor must be considered when treating children in a hyperbaric chamber. Infants may not have the ability to maintain body temperature inside the chamber. Younger patients may have trouble expressing symptoms such as ear pain. Communication with the parents is critical to the child's psychological process. The child may be scared of the chamber. The hyperbaric staff must be able to relate to children.

Situations in which using restraints would be necessary and why

During the course of the technologist's career, he or she may come across a situation in which a patient may be violent and capable of injuring themselves and/or others. In cases such as these, approved restraints may be a necessary precaution. Restraints may also prevent the patient from pulling out intravenous lines or catheters and taking off the grounding bracelet inside the hyperbaric chamber. In the case of restraint use, the technologist must obtain a doctor's order for each event that requires restraining. Carefully explain to the patient, as much as possible, the need for the restraints, and explain each action as you proceed to restrain the patient. Leaving the restraints too loose may allow the patient to loosen themselves while inside the chamber, leaving the restraints too tight may cause the patient to lose circulation in his or her extremities.

Assessing the patient's circulation while restraints are in use

When using restraints on a patient in preparation for a hyperbaric treatment, it is important to assess the patient's circulation before and after the restraints are in place. The circulation is assessed by checking the pulse on the extremity at which point the restraint is placed. The technologist should check the circulation before the use of restraints to assess the strength and quality of the pulses so that he or she will notice a change in the pulses when reassessing them after the restraints are in place. Do not place the restraints directly over the pulse point on any part of the body because you will need to assess the pulse for that extremity. Once you locate the pulse point on each extremity, time the pulse for a full minute, note the quality of the pulse (fast or slow), and note the strength of the pulse (bounding or barely palpable).

Maintaining patient privacy and confidentiality according to HIPAA

Protecting confidential information is very important in our culture of new technology, with more information at our fingertips every day. The HIPAA Privacy Rule controls the input and output of personal patient information. HIPAA stands for the American Health Insurance Portability and Accountability Act of 1996. A HIPAA violation can mean fines and prison time for all those involved. HIPAA applications for hyperbaric facilities are as follows: keeping paper charts closed when not in use; writing initials on the patient board instead of the patient's first and last names; locking the computer screen before walking away; being aware of your surroundings when discussing patients and their care; keeping the patient's physical privacy in mind when opening exam room doors or opening the curtains in the hyperbaric suite; and last but not least, shredding documents with personal patient information instead of discarding them in the trash bins.

Keeping accurate medical records as it pertains to chamber logs and dive profiles

Accurate record keeping in hyperbarics is very important because it not only keeps the patient safe, but it also holds the technologist accountable and protects medical personnel in a court of law. When a technologist signs his or her name on a document, a statement is being made indicating that certain tasks were performed or certain observations were made by that tech. Do not under any circumstances sign your name or initials on something you did not actually do. On the other side of that coin, if it was not signed or written down, it was not done. So be sure to document everything you do! When charting on a permanent medical document, be sure to write legibly so that other medical professionals may be able to read it and follow what was done. To ensure that the records you keep are accurate, double-check your math on the dive profiles and tables and double-check your numbers between the chamber console and the chamber logs.

Infection Control Measures

Key elements of universal precautions for infection control

Universal precautions refer to the use of personal protective equipment for body substance isolation to prevent infection. Infection control is a very important aspect of hyperbaric treatments. Any time multiple patients are being treated in a hyperbaric suite, the prevention of infection by cross-contamination must remain a top priority. It is important to change gloves and/or gowns when switching between patients, even if this takes extra time. Be sure to wash or sanitize your hands as well. Viruses and infections are usually very aggressive in a hospital environment. By taking certain precautions, we may be able to prevent the worsening of the patient's condition. We also safeguard our own health as well as that of our fellow colleagues.

Approved disinfectants for the hyperbaric chamber and equipment

Soap and water and a lint-free cloth may be used to clean the chamber, gurney, sled, mattress, and pillows. Approved disinfectants, such as Tor-HB, STAT III TB, Ascend, LpH se, etc., may also be used. Be sure to use proper personal protective equipment when using any type of chemical cleaner. Chemical concentrates must be diluted with water at the manufacturer's recommended ratios in order to prevent damage to surfaces. The manufacturer's usable shelf life of a diluted chemical cleaning solution is one week, and the container should be labeled accordingly. Do not spray cleaners onto exposed electrical wires or circuits. The interior of the chamber should be cleaned weekly and as needed.

Dangers affiliated with the off-gassing of cleaning chemicals inside the chamber

Some chemical cleaners contain volatile organic compounds (VOCs). These VOCs have a high vapor pressure, which results in a low boiling point at normal room temperature; this means they can easily evaporate. VOCs give off vapors, or they off-gas vapors, into the ambient atmosphere. These vapors are damaging to a patient's health when inhaled. If a hyperbaric chamber is cleaned with a chemical product containing VOCs, the dangerous effects at pressure are hazardous to a patient's health. This is why it is important to only use approved chemical cleaners and to dilute them appropriately according to the manufacturer's instructions.

Proper hand hygiene techniques

Healthcare workers are held to a higher standard when it comes to proper hand hygiene. Not only must healthcare workers strive to keep their hands clean, but they must also keep all surfaces and equipment clean that they touch on a daily basis. Germs spread easily: from door handles, to phones and keyboards. The United States Centers for Disease Control and Prevention recommends washing or sanitizing hands before and after every patient contact. The proper steps for hand washing are as follows: Wet hands under running water, apply soap and lather by rubbing vigorously for at least 20 seconds, rinse hands and use a paper towel or an air dryer to dry, use the towel or an elbow to shut off the water. Healthcare workers should be mindful of covering any open sores or cuts and avoid direct contact of hands with mucous membranes.

Common personal protective equipment

Personal protective equipment (PPE) is required when working with patients. Gloves, gowns, masks, shoe coverings, and face shields are all examples of PPE. Gloves are always worn when working with patients or sterile equipment. Change gloves and sanitize hands before and after every patient contact. Gowns may be used when there is a potential for contact with any fluids from a patient. Masks may be worn in a sterile field, such as surgery, or to protect the healthcare worker's nose when dealing with an odorous wound, or the changing and cleaning of a soiled patient. Shoe coverings are generally used in sterile fields. Face shields may be used when there is potential of coming into contact with patient fluids or when working with chemicals, such as when diluting chemical disinfectants for a cleaning solution.

Chamber Equipment

Routing of the compression gas supply and exhaust

The rules for the piping of gas into a building for hyperbaric chamber use come from the National Fire Protection Association Health Care Facilities Code 99. Gas lines piped inside the building fall under the "Gas and Vacuum Systems" chapter. When the gas pipes pass the zone valve into the hyperbaric suite, the gas lines fall under chapter 14, """Hyperbarics." The gas piped into the building for compression comes either from a liquid oxygen system (monoplace) or an air compressor (multiplace). The gas line in then routed into the chamber. The minimum rate at which the hyperbaric chamber is to be ventilated is three actual cubic feet per minute per each chamber occupant. When the chamber is "on," the gas is vented, or exhausted, into an exhaust pipe that is routed outside of the building, and away from any intakes. What are the quality assurance measures for compression gas supply, and why is it important?

Quality assurance measures for compression gas supply

The liquid oxygen supply for compression of a monoplace chamber must be sampled and tested by the gas supply company. These samples must be tested in a certified laboratory, and the results of the test should be delivered to the hospital maintenance staff and to the hyperbaric technologist with each gas delivery. To pass the quality assurance measures, the gas should be 99.5% pure. The air compressor for compression of a multiplace chamber should be sampled at the intake and downstream from the compressor during the inspection intervals. These samples should be tested at a certified laboratory, and the results should be kept on file in the hyperbaric suite. It is important to measure for quality assurance in order to keep the occupants of the chamber safe and at optimal health. Too many parts per million of a different gas in the mixture could cause equipment problems as well.

Inspection procedures for the compression gas supply pathway

Inspection of the gas supply pathway for a monoplace system is simple compared to a multiplace system. All gas supply lines shall be inspected for unnatural bends, deep scratches, improper fitting placement, and code requirements. The air compressor (multiplace only) shall be inspected for oil leaks and oil-supply levels, intake placement, and possible debris in the intake filter. The gas exhaust for hyperbaric chamber operations shall be located outside of the building, and it should be away from any intakes and building openings, and it should have the proper signage posted, according to the National Fire Protection Association Health Care Facilities Code 99 (No Smoking. Danger: High-Pressure Oxygen Exhaust). The exhaust line shall be inspected for proper placement and possible debris inside the pipe, which could potentially block the gas from exhausting. Monoplace gas lines shall be inspected monthly, and multiplace gas lines shall be inspected on a daily, weekly, monthly, quarterly, and yearly schedule.

General safety practices for liquid oxygen

The following are general safety guidelines for liquid oxygen (LOX): Do not let your skin touch any part of the converter piping. If you have not received training on LOX and the associated equipment, such as valves and regulators, do not attempt to operate any part of the system. NFPA regulations should be followed when storing and using LOX. A copy of the material safety data sheet must be kept on the site. Do not keep hydrocarbons near the converter area. Always wear loose-fitting leather gloves and safety eyewear when operating LOX systems or when touching the converter. Hands, clothing, and tools must be cleaned and free of oils and grease when working around LOX systems.

Breathing gas supply

<u>Connection and operation</u>
The gas breathing supply includes the liquid oxygen system, compressed air tanks, gas lines, regulators, flowmeters, valves, masks, and hoods. When performing the startup checks before the first treatment, the oxygen valve for each chamber must be turned on. The compressed air bottle valves must be turned on. Ensure that the pounds-per-square-inch and pressure measurements are within parameters. Demand masks must be assembled and attached to the chamber port. Nonrebreather masks must be attached to the chamber port. Hoods must be assembled and fitted to the patient, and they must be attached to a chamber port. To replace an empty gas bottle, turn off the valve and bleed the line of gas. Use a wrench to unscrew the regulator. Screw the tank cap over the valve. Mark the bottle as empty and remove from the hyperbaric suite secured to a tank cart.

<u>Quality assurance measures for breathing gas supply</u>
The liquid oxygen (LOX) supply is used not only for compression (monoplace), but also for the breathing gas supply. The LOX is sampled and laboratory tested by the LOX supply company. The results of the testing are delivered along with the LOX to the hyperbaric center, where they are kept on file. The concentration of pure oxygen should never go below 99.5%. The breathing gas supply is a closed system, so that after delivery, there is no opportunity for contamination. If the LOX supply becomes diluted with other gases, such as carbon dioxide, hydrocarbons, or carbon monoxide, the gas quality inside the pressurized chamber decreases, and the patient could be harmed.

<u>Troubleshooting and maintaining the various elements of the breathing gas system</u>
If the hyperbaric chamber does not operate when the master valve is turned on, there are a few troubleshooting techniques the technologist can attempt. Check to see that the main oxygen supply valve and the local chamber oxygen supply valve are in the "on position. These valves are called quarter-turn ball valves. If the handle is parallel to the gas line, then the oxygen supply is flowing freely. If the handle is perpendicular to the gas line, then the oxygen is cut off. Another method of troubleshooting the chamber is to ensure that the chamber door handle is completely closed shut. The door handle may appear shut, but if it is even slightly left ajar, the chamber will not operate.

Type of gas supply used for air breaks

Compressed (high pressure) air in the yellow air tanks are used to give the patients air breaks inside the chamber. The air tank is secured to a rack or a wall, usually with a chain. A regulator is used to reduce the pressure from high (2000–3000 psi) to low (200 psi), and the air flows through the gas line to a flowmeter. A nonrebreather mask is connected to the flowmeter. A demand mask does not require a flowmeter, and it will attach directly to the gas line fed from the regulator. A typical air break schedule for a patient is 30-5-30-5-30, with a few exceptions. The patient must be observed carefully to make sure he or she is using the mask correctly (it is not positioned upside down, it has a tight seal, and the patient is breathing deep enough for the demand mask).

Emergency shut-off procedures in relation to pressure reduction

In the event of a fire inside of the hyperbaric chamber, the technologist may turn off the master valve, secure the oxygen valve, and then press and hold down the emergency vent/exhaust button. This event is the only time the technologist is allowed to emergency vent the chamber with a patient inside. The emergency vent/exhaust button is tested weekly for optimal operational efficiency. In the event of a fire outside of the chamber, the technologist may depressurize the chamber at a faster rate with direction from a hyperbaric physician. The location of the fire must be known, and it must be determined if the fire poses a threat to the hyperbaric center. After the chamber is on the surface, evacuate the patient and secure the oxygen valve at the chamber. The main oxygen valve should be secured only after all patients are safely evacuated from the chamber.

Purpose of a regulator

High-pressure gas coming from a liquid oxygen tank or a cylinder is too high to be useful in a clinical setting. A regulator controls the pressure and reduces it for patient use. Regulators are designed to handle high pressures, but they are also designed to carry only specific gases. Regulators may be installed as part of a gas manifold system, or they may be installed directly onto the cylinder. A regulator allows the hyperbaric technologist to control the amount of oxygen or air delivered to the patient through a demand valve mask, a nasal cannula, a hood, or a nonrebreather mask. The air cylinder (yellow) pressure for hyperbaric air break use is typically 2000–3000 psi, and it is fed into a regulator that reduces the pressure to 40–70 psi; typically, the pressure is then further reduced by a flowmeter to 1–6 psi. A regulator attached to an oxygen tank (green) reduces the pressure to 0.5–25 psi for patient use.

Regulator vs. flowmeter

A regulator reduces the gas pressure from high-pressure cylinders or liquid oxygen tanks into breathable gas pressure for patient use. A flowmeter is attached down the line from the regulator for the purpose of adjusting the amount of gas pressure in pounds per square inch (psi) that the patient breathes in. A flowmeter may or may not be attached depending on the gas line system. The flowmeter may convert the gas pressure down to 1–6 psi, whereas a regulator may convert the high-pressure gas to 40–70 psi. Inside a hyperbaric chamber, the regulator may be used for a demand valve mask, meaning that the gas will only flow when the patient breathes in. A nonrebreather mask, or a nasal cannula, is typically attached to a flowmeter for a free flow, meaning that the gas flows freely whether the patient takes a breath or not. If the hyperbaric patient has a tough time taking a deep enough breath for the demand mask, the technologist may switch to a free-flow mask option.

Fire extinguishing system, how to activate it for a multiplace chamber

The preferred method for extinguishing fires inside the multiplace hyperbaric chamber is through the spray of water. This waterspray is accomplished through the use of a system of deluge nozzles dispersed intermittently throughout the hyperbaric multiplace chamber. The waterspray issuing forth from these nozzles must be a fine mist and an even spray. The waterspray deluge system is activated by the chamber operator by use of a button on the chamber console outside of the chamber. Handlines may be used by the chamber inside tenders. Handlines are located in strategic areas inside the chamber and are activated by a quarter-turn ball valve.

Activation of the fire alarm for the hyperbaric facility

If there is a fire in the hyperbaric suite or facility, the fire must be called in to either EMS (outpatient facility), or to the hospital's emergency code (facility inside a hospital). The emergency code is usually posted on every hospital telephone. The hospital usually will provide a list of emergency codes to be worn with the employee's badge. When calling in to report a fire, have as much information about the fire as possible: fire location, fire severity, if any staff or patients are in danger, and smoke quality. After the code is called in, the fire pull handle should be pulled. All personnel should be located and informed that this alarm is not a drill.

Operating each component of the facility fire extinguishing system

The majority of fire extinguishers generally operate in the same fashion. The hyperbaric technologist must know the location of each fire extinguisher and fire pull alarm. Fire extinguishers may be operated using the following acronym: PASS, which stands for pull, aim, squeeze, and sweep. After taking the fire extinguisher from its mounted position, pull the locking pin out of the handle. Aim the extinguisher hose at the base of the fire. Squeeze the trigger handle while holding the bottle firmly. Sweep the extinguisher slowly from one side of the fire to the other, and repeat until help comes or until the extinguisher runs out. If there is imminent danger to your person, flee the vicinity of the fire.

Proceeding with emergency operations during a fire

Emergency steps to follow during a hyperbaric facility fire include: confirmation of the fire, call in the fire code, bring the hyperbaric chambers to the surface, evacuate the patients, and shut off the oxygen valves. General fire procedures may be accomplished by the following acronym: RACE, which stands for rescue, alarm, contain, and extinguish. When a fire alarm is sounded or a fire has been confirmed, the technologist must attempt to rescue all patients and direct them to a safe location. If the alarm has not been sounded, the technologist must call in the fire code at this time. All staff must attempt to contain the fire by closing all doors and storing away all equipment. Lastly, the technologist must attempt to extinguish the fire using the fire extinguisher. The hyperbaric staff must act as a cohesive team during any emergency.

Typical communication system inside a hyperbaric chamber

The hyperbaric chamber will have a communications system installed. The communication system outside of the chamber ends in a handset for the chamber operator. The chamber operator will be able to control the volume the patient hears, as well as the operator volume. The communication system inside of the chamber is typically an "open mic" system. The chamber operator is able to hear conversations and noises on the inside of the chamber through the use of the open microphone system. In the multiplace chamber, the inside tender may be equipped with a microphone and headset. This microphone will also be open mic to eliminate the electric arc when the mic button is pushed. A small hole may be in both ear speakers of the headset in order to prevent a face squeeze during travel to pressure.

Voice and visual communications between the patient and the chamber operator

Voice and visual communications between the hyperbaric chamber operator and the chamber occupant are vitally important. Every effort must be made to have a clear, understandable communication system. The chamber operator must speak slowly and clearly, and he or she must listen to the patient's concerns and be able to decipher them. If the operator does not speak the patient's language, a system of flashcards must be devised and kept on hand. The operator may also be able to learn and use a few key words and phrases in the patient's language. Alternately, the operator and patient may develop a system of hand signals over time to be able to communicate effectively and efficiently. If there is any doubt as to clarity in communication, an interpreter must be called.

Complication in communications between the patient and the chamber operator

From time to time during the course of hyperbaric treatments, the patient and operator may lose the ability to communicate through the communications system. If this happens, flashcards that explain pertinent information must be crafted and kept on hand. If the patient cannot read, a careful system of hand signals may be used to put the patient at ease while bringing the chamber to the surface if necessary. If the patient indicates that he or she can no longer hear the entertainment system during the compression phase, the operator may advise the patient either loudly or through hand signals to try the maneuvers for clearing the ears. If the patient uses sign language, a visual line of sight to a laptop computer will be essential for interpreter communications.

Chamber Operations

Hyperbaric chamber standard operating procedures

Hyperbaric oxygen chamber operations require standard operating procedures. The patient must be appropriately attired, examined physically for contraband, and educated regarding the dangers prior to placement onto the hyperbaric stretcher. The patient may require a transfer onto the hyperbaric gurney. Insert the hyperbaric gurney attachments into the rail sockets and lock the gurney. To release the sled from the gurney, pull up on the latch at the head and push the sled forward. Roll the sled into the chamber until the latch catches once seated into the chamber. Attach the patient grounding cord to the chamber ground socket. Release the lock on the gurney, and roll the gurney to a proper distance away from the chamber. Check that the supply pressure is present, then close and lock the chamber door. Turn on the master control valve, and turn the pressure set to the proper treatment pressure. Be sure to set the rate for patient comfort. Once the chamber reaches the prescribed treatment pressure, start the timer.

Inspecting a control console for the chamber

All indicators on the hyperbaric chamber control console must be operating properly before patient treatment can be initiated. If the hyperbaric chamber has an electronic control system, the chamber console will automatically perform a self-test every time it is turned on. This will typically cause an audible alarm to sound. If the self-test in executed correctly, the controls will adjust themselves to the default settings. For a manual control console, an inspection is performed by turning on the master control valve and turning the pressure set knob to idle pressure. The gauges are functioning properly when the needles on both the pressure set gauge and the chamber pressure gauge are moving accordingly. Check to see if the supply pressure indicator and the chamber pressure indicator are both showing a positive pressure measurement. The communication function is inspected by turning on the master control valve and talking through the mouthpiece.

Manual vs. automatic controls for hyperbaric chambers

Hyperbaric chambers use a variety of controls for operation. Generally, these controls can be categorized into two types: manual and automatic. An automatic control chamber uses an electronic system. In this automatic console, the pressure set, rate set, chamber cycles, chamber pressure, and temperature are all in a digital format. When the master control valve is switched on, the chamber pressure, pressure set, and rate set will automatically be set to default, which is typically 1.5 psi. A manual control system uses knobs and pressure gauges to operate the chamber. There are two pressure gauges on a manual console: One gauge is the actual chamber pressure, and the other gauge is the pressure the operator may set for the pressure treatment. When the master valve is switched on, the default is 0 psi until the operator increases the pressure set gauge by turning the pressure set knob.

Functions of the console controls for automatic chamber operation

The automatic control system for the hyperbaric chamber is called the electronic control module (ECM). On the ECM is the master control valve, which has three modes: vent, off, and on. The vent setting is used to emergency vent the pressurized chamber. The gas supply to the chamber is absent when the master control valve is set to off. The emergency vent button may be used during specified crisis situations and should be tested once a week. In order to decompress the chamber emergently, the master control valve must be set to vent and the emergency vent button should be held down until the ECM shuts off. This usually happens in 90 seconds. The pressure set knob is used to set the chamber pressure to the desired depth. The rate set knob is used to set the rate at which the chamber travels to and from pressure.

Specific situations for which chamber emergency procedures are designed to address

Situations requiring urgent operator attention and adherence to protocol include chamber or ancillary equipment malfunctions, gas or air supply issues, and patient health emergencies. In certain manufacturers' chambers, such as Sechrist, when the chamber pressure is lost or the electronic system fails, there are backups in place that will put the chamber in a "safe state." In this case, the chamber will automatically decompress at a slow rate. The rate may be adjusted by turning the purge/ventilation flow control valve up or down. If there is an uncontrollable increase in pressure, turn off the master control valve and shut off the chamber gas supply valve. If an oxygen leak is detected, correct it if possible, or proceed with aborting the treatment. During a loss of communications, use flashcards or hand signals to communicate with the patient and determine if the treatment needs to be aborted. For a stuck door-locking pin, stick a blunt object inside the lock pinhole to release the pin. Deterioration of the patient's physical or mental condition requires specific steps depending on the emergency as well as informing the attending physician and nurse.

Areas covered by an ideal safety program to ensure emergency preparedness

Hyperbaric oxygen technicians should be familiar with all emergency chamber procedures. Incorporate the practice of handling mock crisis scenarios to help ensure proper response and general preparedness. For a patient seizure incident, a suspected pneumothorax, an unresponsive or cardiac arrest patient, or an incapacitated chamber operator, you must stop all chamber travel and call the hyperbaric physician. If the emergency can be resolved or it is a false alarm, the hyperbaric physician may direct the technologist to resume the chamber treatment. If it is a life-threatening emergency, wait until the patient resumes breathing, and abort the treatment by decompressing the chamber at a rate that is dictated by the hyperbaric physician. An emergency response team may need to be activated. Be sure to switch the patient's bed and linens in case of the use of a defibrillator. Emergency procedures for commonly identified scenarios should be memorized by all of the hyperbaric staff.

Inspection procedure for the emergency vent in a chamber

In the event of a fire inside of the chamber, the hyperbaric technologist may use the emergency vent/exhaust button to bring the chamber to the surface in less than two minutes. Therefore, it is critical that the emergency vent/exhaust button or switch be inspected frequently. The typical schedule is weekly, semiannually, and annually. The semiannual and annual tests are completed by a certified chamber technician for the type of chamber requiring inspection. The weekly tests may be completed by the chamber operator/hyperbaric technologist on staff at the facility. For the weekly test of a general chamber type, close and lock the chamber door and pressurize the chamber to 2 atmospheres absolute (ATA). Open and close the compression valve to both extremes to determine the high and low liters per minute. Then, pressurize the chamber to 3 ATA and wait the designated time for the chamber to be completely filled with 100% oxygen (usually 12 minutes for an average-sized monoplace chamber). Turn the master valve to the "vent" position, and then press and hold the emergency vent button. Use a timer to determine if the chamber completes the vent in less than two minutes.

Various treatment tables and decision criteria used for decompression

The *U.S. Navy Diving Manual* has standardized dive tables used for decompression sickness (types I and II), arterial gas embolism, carbon monoxide poisoning, and gas gangrene, etc. The relevant and most used treatment tables are 5, 6, and 6A. Table 5 has a descent rate of 20 feet per minute (fpm), and it has an ascent rate of 1 fpm while breathing 100% oxygen. Oxygen breathing time starts when the diver reaches 60 feet and continues for one period, or 20 minutes followed by a 5-minute air break. The diver breathes oxygen for another 20 minutes before the ascent starts. The total treatment time not including descent is 135 minutes. Treatment table 6 follows the same rules as treatment table 5. Table 6 may be extended, if needed, for two periods at 60 feet and two periods at 30 feet. The total treatment time for table 6 is 285 minutes. Treatment table 6A follows the same rules as well, but it goes to a depth of 165 feet, and it has a total treatment time of 350 minutes.

Decompression procedures for the hyperbaric chamber

The hyperbaric oxygen chamber has strict operating procedures including decompression procedures. Decompression for monoplace chambers generally includes bringing the chamber to the surface at a rate of 1.5 psi/minute, which may be raised to 2.5 psi/minute if the patient can tolerate it and has no lung problems. Decompression procedures are the same for a multiplace chamber except when used for treatments such as decompression sickness and arterial gas embolism. In these cases, the *U.S. Navy Diving Manual* decompression tables and treatment tables are used. The treatment table ascent rate is 1 fpm, and the decompression table ascent rate is 60 fpm. The Navy's decompression tables take into account the uptake and elimination of nitrogen; therefore, there are timed decompression stops to allow the nitrogen bubbles the adequate time needed to dissolve into the bloodstream. These decompression tables are based on studies done by John Scott Haldane in the 1900s on body compartment decompression half-times.

Conditions that typically lead to decompression sickness in tenders

The tenders inside multiplace hyperbaric chambers are susceptible to decompression sickness. Dalton's law tells us that the partial pressures of all inhaled gases are increased as the total pressure is increased. Henry's law tells us that the amount of nitrogen that can be dissolved into the tissues is directly proportional to the nitrogen partial pressure. The amount of nitrogen is not evenly distributed between all body tissues. Nitrogen distribution depends on body fat and the perfusion of blood. Therefore, nitrogen can form bubbles in different parts of the body if the atmospheric pressure is lowered faster than the body can dissolve the nitrogen out of solution. In hyperbaric-chamber terms, if the chamber is decompressed too quickly, the inside tender may suffer decompression sickness. The tender can benefit from periods of breathing 100% oxygen during the dive because the nitrogen half-life will be eliminated faster.

U.S. Navy Diving Manual standard air decompression table computations

The *U.S. Navy Diving Manual* decompression tables are applied to air breathing at greater than sea level pressures. When breathing air under pressure, the body takes on additional nitrogen, and that may cause decompression sickness. The nitrogen must be monitored in order to decompress safely. The depth and the total bottom time can determine how much nitrogen has been added to the body. The "no-decompression" table has letters assigned to a dive to determine the "residual nitrogen time" on the surface before a second dive. If the surface time is 12 hours or more, the dive is not considered repetitive. The standard air decompression tables are used when a diver needs to make decompression stops to off-gas nitrogen. For example, if a diver makes a dive to 80 feet for 80 minutes, the 80-ft. table states that the diver would have to stop at 20 feet for 2 minutes and again at 10 feet for 31 minutes. These tables also use letters for the residual nitrogen time.

Creating a dive profile for the inside tender versus the patient

The tender inside the multiplace hyperbaric oxygen chamber is accountable for patient safety as well as his or her own personal health and well-being. Tenders should keep a dive log with dive profiles to track the residual nitrogen time between dives in order to avoid decompression sickness. When a body is pressurized in a chamber, the partial pressures of the gases that are inhaled increase because the total pressure of the atmosphere is increased. The amount of nitrogen uptake is increased, and the body will continue to store nitrogen for the duration of the chamber treatment. When the chamber is decompressed, some of the nitrogen inside the tender's body will diffuse into the blood, pass into the lungs, and be exhaled out of the body. The remaining nitrogen may form bubbles if the chamber is decompressed faster than the body can compensate. The tender must keep in mind that he or she should not fly in an airplane at least 12 hours before and after a dive.

FDA-approved indications in order to initiate hyperbaric oxygen therapy protocols

The accepted emergency indications for hyperbaric oxygen therapy (HBOT) approved by the Food and Drug Administration are acute carbon monoxide poisoning, gas gangrene, acute brain injury (severe cranial injury), acute spinal disorders, acute arterial circulatory disturbance, decompression sickness, air or gas embolism, severe burn and cold injuries, retinal artery obstruction, ileus, and acute myocardial infarction. The accepted nonemergency indications are as follows: chronic carbon monoxide poisoning, chronic circulatory disturbance with peripheral refractory ulcer, ischemic skin pedicle after skin graft, sudden deafness, chronic refractory osteomyelitis, radiation ulcer, motor paresis, refractory spinal cord neuropathy, and cancer therapy associated with radiation injury. The HBOT patient diagnosis will fall under these indications.

Hyperbaric dive profile of a typical patient

There are a few protocols for the hyperbaric oxygen patient diving in a wound-care facility chamber. Each indication has its own rationale for treatment in a hyperbaric chamber and the type of dive profile desired. Patients with diabetic foot ulcers, for example, dive at 2 atmospheres absolute (ATA) for 90 minutes while breathing 100% oxygen with no air breaks. The 2-ATA dive profile might be as follows: Leave the surface at 0800, reach the bottom at 0810, leave the bottom at 0940, reach the surface at 0950, for a total of 110 minutes. Patients with a radiation injury, chronic refractory osteomyelitis, or necrotizing fasciitis, for example, dive at 2.5 ATA for 90 minutes while breathing 100% oxygen with two 5-minute air breaks. The 2.5-ATA dive profile might be as follows: Leave the surface at 0800, reach the bottom at 0815, air break begins at 0845, air break ends at 0850, air break begins at 0920, air break ends at 0925, leave the bottom at 0955, reach the surface at 1010, for a total of 130 minutes.

Effects that pressure could have on ancillary equipment and supplies

When a hyperbaric chamber is pressurized, the pressure may have an effect on the ancillary equipment and supplies used inside the chamber. Some examples of ancillary equipment are the transcutaneous oxygen monitor (TCOM), mechanical ventilator, and IV pump; catheters, injectors, and tracheostomy tubes are examples of supplies. The TCOM is placed outside of the chamber and is fed information through the leads attached to the portholes in the chamber door. A mechanical ventilator requires constant over bottom pressure, respiratory staff in attendance, and a depth conversion chart. It consumes 0.3 actual cubic feet per minute. An intravenous pump requires a special high-pressure pump with constant over bottom pressure and special hard tubing. The catheter, injector, and tracheostomy tubes are all examples of air spaces that need to be either filled with fluid or eliminated. According to the National Fire Protection Association, the safety director has the authority to limit or restrict any item deemed to be unsafe or hazardous.

Specifications for the chamber exhaust

The gas (oxygen) exhaust for the hyperbaric oxygen chamber must be located outside the building in the open air. The gas exhaust pipes must not be within any type of enclosure. Once the master valve on a hyperbaric chamber is opened, the gas supply will vent into the chamber at the patient's head and exhaust out of the chamber at the patient's feet. The gas exhaust will then flow as directly as possible out of the facility. Approximately 36,000 liters of oxygen will be pumped out of the exhaust pipes per treatment. The chamber gas exhaust must not be placed within a main thoroughfare. The area for the exhaust should have legible signs stating a warning for the presence of oxygen. The exhaust pipes should either be facing down or facing up with a guard for debris in place.

Material safety data sheets

Material safety data sheets (MSDSs) should be readily available in the hyperbaric and wound care center. Some facilities will have them in a binder stored in a well-known area, and some facilities have their MSDSs in digital form on a computer desktop. The facility is required to have MSDSs on all chemicals and gases used in the facility. The MSDSs should contain the following information: chemical content, reactivity to other chemicals, flammability, and other hazards related to the product. Every facility is required to keep its own MSDSs current and up to date. Examples of items in hyperbaric facilities requiring an MSDS are oxygen, air, alcohol prep pads, TOR-HB cleaning solution, wound care medicines and dressings, and soaps. MSDSs can be found on most products' websites or on the website for the Occupational Safety and Health Administration.

Material analysis form

The material analysis form in hyperbaric operations is used to approve or prohibit items that cannot be easily removed from the patient once inside a hyperbaric chamber. Examples would be pacemakers, joint replacements, internal plates, pain medication pumps, or weaves. Prior to treatment, the first lists to be consulted are the prohibited items and the approved items. Also to be considered is the experience of other hyperbaric oxygen centers that might have had to approve or prohibit certain items. The material analysis form, or a similar document, is to be approved and signed by the hyperbaric safety director and the medical director. When approval or prohibition is pending, considerations should be made for the flammability of the material, susceptibility to chemical oxidation, the amount of off-gassing, production of static electricity, linen material, and chamber ventilation. The conditions of the approval or prohibition and the reason for the analysis should be noted on the form.

Type of lubrication approved for use in a hyperbaric chamber

Lubricants for use in hyperbaric oxygen chambers must be deemed oxygen safe, or approved for use in pure oxygen environments. Emollients applied in or around oxygen environments should be used sparingly because the lubrication properties are based on the film of the lubricant. Therefore, any excess should be wiped off with a lint-free cloth or paper. Emollients are typically easily ignitable and vulnerable in pressure systems. Lubricants such as Krytox must be safe in both high- and low-pressure systems. They must be nontoxic and nonreactive with standard O-ring materials, aluminum, steel, brass, nylon, and Teflon. Teflon itself is also a lubricant. The lubricant should provide protection from corrosion, and it should be easy to use. Packaging should consist of clearly labeled, individual, sealable, oxygen-clean containers that keep out dirt and dust.

Type of signage used around the oxygen supply and high-pressure medical air supply

Cautionary or instructional signs and labels used for the purposes of hyperbaric oxygen operations are very important. Staff or vendors working near any high-pressure gases require knowledge of safety and a general awareness of the surroundings. Patients and visitors should also be aware of safety concerns. Areas in which high-pressure signage is required are around the yellow air tank storage, air tank usage, and high-pressure wall unit. The high-pressure warning sign should be yellow, and it should read "High-Pressure Medical Air." Oxygen is a very dangerous gas to work with, especially under high-pressure conditions. When working with oxygen, do not use open flames and do not smoke. Oxygen itself is not flammable, but when a flame ignites in the vicinity, an explosion may occur. The color for oxygen signage is green, and the oxygen supply warning sign should read "HBO Chamber Oxygen Supply Valve." The oxygen exhaust warning sign outside the building should read "Danger: Oxygen Exhaust. Positively No Smoking or Open Flame within 25 Feet."

Verification of the continuity of the patient and facility grounding assembly

The grounding assembly for the patient ground and the facility ground should be inspected and tested once a week, or testing can be performed more often if damage is suspected. The compliance range for the facility ground to the chamber must be less than 1 ohm, and the compliance range for the patient grounding assembly must be between 0.950 and 1.050 M ohms. A multimeter is used to measure these values. The patient grounding cord should be measured from end to end. The facility ground must be measured from the chamber ground port to the facility ground (usually located on the wall behind the chamber) using a connector cord with the multimeter.

Ideal temperature range of the hyperbaric treatment room

The ideal temperature range of the hyperbaric treatment room is between 70 and 80° Fahrenheit according to the National Fire Protection Association Health Care Facilities Code 99 (NFPA 99). This is important to the patient's comfort level during hyperbaric treatments and for keeping the hyperbaric and ancillary equipment cool. The multiplace chamber may have in place for patient comfort an air conditioning system by the circulating of ambient air inside the chamber over coils that contain a mixture of water and glycol. Warm or cold water may flow inside the coils to produce warm or cool air inside the chamber. Humidification and dehumidification are also allowed per NFPA 99.

Purpose of keeping the chamber free of dust and lint

The hyperbaric oxygen chamber interior and exterior should not only be kept clean, but it also should be kept free of dust and lint to prevent clogging of vents and piping and to keep it at an optimal operational status. If a chamber has to be taken out of service for even a day for a clogged exhaust vent filter, it could cost the company or facility thousands of dollars. A clogged exhaust vent filter screen is also dangerous to the hyperbaric patient currently being treated because it may cause the atmosphere inside the chamber to become contaminated. To clean the exhaust vent filter screen, use a screwdriver to detach it from the chamber and soak it in water for 10 minutes. Once the soaking is complete, carefully blow compressed air through the screen until it is dry, then reinstall.

Thoroughly inspecting patients prior to insertion into the chamber

The inspection process for patients prior to a hyperbaric treatment may vary depending on the type of patient, but the same safety elements need to be in place. If the patient speaks the language of the technologist, walks without help to the treatment room, and understands the hyperbaric process well enough, the technologist may only ask the pretreatment checklist questions prior to entering the chamber. On the other hand, if the patient comes in on a hospital bed, does not walk, does not understand the technologist's language, and is apathetic toward the treatment, the technologist may decide to undress the patient and thoroughly check him or her for contraband, and even wash parts of the patient's body to remove oils or prohibited substances prior to insertion into the chamber. The pretreatment process depends on the hyperbaric technologist's discretion, but safety should never be compromised.

Communication with a patient who does not speak your language inside the chamber

Communication between the hyperbaric patient and the hyperbaric technologist is imperative to proper chamber operations. If the hyperbaric patient does not speak the language of the technologist or if the patient is deaf or otherwise impaired, other forms of communication must be used. Alternate forms of communication can be sign language, hand signals, interpreters, and flashcards. The technologist may attempt to learn a few key words and phrases in the patient's language and develop a series of hand signals with the patient before initiating hyperbaric oxygen therapy. Using an interpreter for a non-English-speaking patient is the best option for communication. Flashcards in the patient's language should be kept available to the technologist and to the patient before, during, and after the hyperbaric treatment.

Nutritional information for hyperbaric and wound care patients

Nutritional information regarding protein, caloric intake, and vitamins/minerals may help the patient to recover faster from wounds while he or she is undergoing hyperbaric oxygen treatment. If the patient is deficient in protein, it may delay healing by prolonging the inflammatory response. It may also cause edema to spread. On the other hand, adequate protein intake can help with wound healing by producing collagen synthesis. If the patient does not have an adequate caloric intake, catabolism (protein is broken down for energy instead of carbohydrates) is promoted and wound healing is adversely affected. Vitamin A may help to reduce inflammation, increase collagen synthesis, and limit infection. Vitamin C also plays a role in collagen synthesis, and it may decrease infection through leukocyte activation. Zinc also helps collagen synthesis and increases wound strength. Vitamin E may decrease the risk of oxygen toxicity and should be taken on a daily basis during the course of hyperbaric oxygen treatments.

Transferring the patient into and out of the hyperbaric chamber

The hyperbaric patient must be loaded into and out of the hyperbaric chamber. In a multiplace chamber, the patient may walk in and sit on a chair where they may receive oxygen via a hood, or they may be placed on a stretcher and wheeled inside the chamber. In a monoplace chamber, the patient must lie on a stretcher and be rolled into the chamber, where they receive oxygen just by breathing in the surrounding atmosphere. The patient must be supine and covered with blankets to his or her preference. The patient's head must be raised to a comfortable position but not too high because this may block the gas flow over the patient or the patient may get too warm. To load the patient, attach the gurney to the chamber, lock the gurney, release the latch, roll the sled into the chamber, and plug in the patient grounding cord. To unload the patient, unplug the patient grounding cord, release the latch, and slide the sled out of the chamber.

Risk factors for inadequate hyperbaric patient preparation

Patients must be adequately prepared for treatment in a hyperbaric chamber. Sufficient preparation includes hyperbaric oxygen orientation and education, changing into the appropriate attire for oxygen treatments, and verifying each item on the patient safety checklist. If the patient did not receive the proper education, he or she might unknowingly bring or wear a prohibited item inside of the hyperbaric chamber, causing a major safety violation. If the patient's attire is not 100% cotton, or a 51% cotton/polyester mix, this poses a fire hazard. If the technician and the patient do not verify each item on the checklist, contraband may be missed and pose a fire hazard or health hazard inside the hyperbaric chamber. Safety should be the number-one priority when working in, with, or around oxygen pressure systems. Be vigilant to make sure you do not get complacent with the day-to-day routines of hyperbaric operations. Following a standard preparation process is important to adhere to for every treatment even with recurrent patients.

Potential sources of ignition inside the chamber

Controlling the potential of a fire inside the hyperbaric oxygen chamber is done by means of eliminating possible sources of ignition. "Ignition" is defined as any energy release that may raise the temperature above the potential energy required to activate a combustion reaction. There are many possible sources of ignition in a hyperbaric oxygen environment: sparks or arcs from electronic devices, electrical heat overload or wire overload, a failed or locked motor, a spark of friction or impact, electrostatic spark, open flames, hot surfaces, preheated items introduced into the chamber, hand warmers, and shock waves. The ignition temperature is also called the autogenous ignition temperature (AIT), and it is used to measure parameters for how individual materials will potentially ignite. During at AIT test, the material is heated until the vapors ignite without an external ignition source. The AIT scale typically decreases with increased oxygen and pressure.

Preventing electric shock

Electric shock occurs when a person comes in contact with two electrical conductors that have different potentials of voltage. The ground or a damp floor is generally a good conductor. The difference of voltage, the time of conductor contact, and the amount and frequency of current are all factors for the magnitude of shock. Grounding is an important aspect of electrical system maintenance. The ability to ground something depends on three things: a ground, a grounded object, and a ground path. To prevent electric shock in a hyperbaric oxygen chamber, the chamber is grounded to the facility, the patient stretcher is grounded to the chamber by use of metallic strips on the bottom of the sled, and the patient is grounded to the stretcher by use of a metal wrist bracelet with a cord that is attached to the chamber.

Flame speed and burn rate of common materials approved for chamber use

Two factors that should be considered when introducing new material into the hyperbaric oxygen chamber are the flame speed and the burn rate of those materials. The flame speed is the rate at which a fire develops, and the burn rate is the rate at which material is consumed and heat is released. Knowledge of these elements is essential for fire control. The flame speed and burn rate are always higher in oxygen than in air. The flame spread rate is calculated in millimeters per second (mm/s). For example, lip balm does not ignite in air, but in oxygen the rate is 46.23 mm/s. The rate for rubber tubing in air is 0.76 mm/s, while in oxygen the rate is 6.096 mm/s. A cotton shirt will not sustain a propagation of a flame in air, but in oxygen, the rate the cloth will burn is 38.1 mm/s.

Temperature parameters for electrical equipment installed in the chamber

The "Hyperbaric" chapter (chapter 14) in NFPA 99 has specific parameters for the temperatures of electrical equipment operating inside a multiplace hyperbaric chamber. The highest operating temperature of any installed electrical equipment inside a hyperbaric chamber should be 85° Celsius, or 185° Fahrenheit. This includes patient monitoring leads and electromedical equipment, such as IV pumps. Exposed live electrical parts are not permitted inside the hyperbaric chamber unless they are certified to be intrinsically safe. The circuit design of headset cables, sensor leads, alarms, etc. should be no more than 28 volts and 0.5 amps.

Ensuring that the pressure is completely equalized before opening the chamber door

Pressure equalization is important in the prevention of barotrauma. The quick evacuation of the oxygen pressure inside a hyperbaric oxygen chamber may lead to barotraumas such as blowing a hole in the eardrum or even a pneumothorax in a patient with lung disease. For this reason, it is important to wait a couple extra minutes for complete chamber pressure to atmospheric pressure equalization. Pressure equalization may be verified by checking the "chamber pressurized" window/indicator on the chamber control console. When the pressure indicator is completely black (the typical color for complete depressurization on most chamber models), unlock the chamber door and open the chamber as soon as possible because there is no gas flow present inside the chamber at this time. Older chamber models have a door design without a lock. The door is affixed by the internal pressure of the chamber.

Typical pressure rate for a hyperbaric treatment

When a patient is treated inside a hyperbaric oxygen chamber, the treatment is set to a certain depth determined by the hyperbaric physician, and this is dependent on the patient's diagnosis. This depth is called the chamber pressure. The hyperbaric technologist may travel the patient to that depth by turning the "pressure set" knob to the desired chamber pressure. The rate at which the patient is traveled to the desired chamber pressure is controlled by the "rate set" knob. The typical default rate set for a hyperbaric chamber with an electronic control system is 1.5 pounds per square inch (psi)/minute. A manual system on a hyperbaric chamber does not have a default. The rate must be set by turning a valve. During a patient's first hyperbaric treatment, it is prudent to drop the rate set to 1.0 psi/minute to prevent barotrauma until the patient is accustomed to the pressure changes.

Two phases of a seizure and when it is appropriate to decompress the chamber

The two phases of an oxygen toxicity seizure are the tonic and clonic phases. During the first phase, known as tonic, the patient is not breathing, so it is extremely important to stop all chamber travel. The second phase, called clonic, may be accompanied by an episode of violent shaking and twitching of the body, and it could last up to two minutes. During this phase, the hyperbaric physician and nurse must be notified immediately. The patient will start the seizure activity and begin to breathe again (although breathing may be irregular). At this point, and under hyperbaric physician supervision, the technologist may decompress the chamber. The emergency response team should already be activated and ready to take over when the chamber is on the surface, the patient is evacuated, and transfer to a nonhyperbaric stretcher has been accomplished.

Possible complications if a patient is not breathing properly during decompression

If the hyperbaric patient does not breathe during the decompression phase of the hyperbaric treatment, the patient will develop barotrauma to the lungs. The signs and symptoms of barotrauma to the lungs include pain to the chest or upper back, difficulty breathing, pale or bluish skin, tracheal shift, and increased anxiety. Spontaneous pneumothorax, mediastinal or subcutaneous emphysema, and arterial gas embolism are all types of lung barotrauma. Treatment of lung barotrauma involves hyperbaric physician notification, recompression, chest tube insertion, and chest X-ray to determine proper placement. Patients must be monitored for an appropriate interval and reevaluated before hyperbaric oxygen treatments can resume.

Safety mechanisms and procedures for securing all chamber openings

In order to pressurize a hyperbaric oxygen chamber, the chamber door must be secured and airtight (and gastight). For older hyperbaric chamber models, the chamber door is secured tight to the chamber by the internal pressure of the chamber. If the chamber has two compartments, the internal chamber door is secured in the same fashion. For newer chamber models, the chamber is secured by a door-locking handle and mechanism. If there are two compartments, such as with a typical multiplace chamber, the door is operated in the same fashion. Some chambers have a safety mechanism in the chamber door called a locking pin. The locking pin engages as the chamber is pressurized past a certain point, typically at 1.5 psi. Functional operation of the locking pin must be observed as part of the weekly chamber test and checklist.

Patient Assessment

Steps conducted during an initial patient consultation

A patient's first visit to a wound care facility should include physician mention of hyperbaric oxygen therapy (HBOT) as a potential treatment course where applicable. Ideally, the doctor would provide thorough education on how HBOT may benefit the patient's condition in conjunction with other healing methods. If it is determined that the patient is a hyperbaric candidate, the physician should impress upon the patient the importance of pressurized oxygen for their condition, and a technician should be brought in to orient the patient on the HBOT process. There should be an emphasis on patient commitment to a complete course of hyperbaric treatments. If possible, the patient should tour the hyperbaric suite to be introduced to the medical staff and to view the chambers and surroundings. This will help ensure the patient's comfort during their first treatment.

Undersea Hyperbaric and Medical Society-approved conditions for patient referral

The Undersea Hyperbaric and Medical Society has its own approved indications for hyperbaric oxygen therapy (HBOT), which include the following: air or gas embolism, carbon monoxide poisoning, clostridial myositis and myonecrosis (gas gangrene), crush injury, compartment syndrome and other acute traumatic ischemias, decompression sickness, arterial insufficiencies, severe anemia, intracranial abscess, necrotizing soft tissue infections, osteomyelitis (refractory), delayed radiation injury (soft-tissue and bony necrosis), compromised grafts and flaps, acute thermal burn injury, and idiopathic sudden sensorineural hearing loss (approved in 2011). Some indications for HBOT are considered the primary treatment modality, whereas other indications are considered adjunctive, or secondary, to surgery or other pharmacologic considerations. Decompression sickness and air or gas embolism are examples of primary indications for HBOT. Some examples of adjunctive indications are compromised graft or flap, crush injury, acute thermal burn injury, and delayed radiation injury.

Typical roles within a hyperbaric clinical team and their responsibilities

For hyperbaric operations to run at top efficiency, all team members must collaborate and diligently perform their roles. First and foremost, to run a hyperbaric oxygen chamber, a certified hyperbaric technologist is needed. The hyperbaric technologist must have been certified previously in a healthcare-related field, such as emergency medical technician, or licensed practical nurse/licensed vocational nurse. The hyperbaric technologist not only operates the hyperbaric chambers, but also educates and prepares the patient for treatment. The hyperbaric safety director is responsible for all safety aspects of hyperbaric operations and maintenance schedules. The certified hyperbaric registered nurse is responsible for the well-being of the patients, delivery of medications upon doctor orders, and wound care. The hyperbaric medical director is responsible for making the ultimate decisions regarding patient treatment inside a hyperbaric oxygen chamber. These team members must cohesively work together in order to achieve optimal patient healing rates.

Potential benefits of hyperbaric oxygen therapy

The benefits of the increased pressurized oxygen used in hyperbaric oxygen therapy are many. The increased pressure inside the hyperbaric chamber causes vasoconstriction of the blood vessels, thereby lowering edema. The oxygen at 100% overloads the red blood cells (hemoglobin) and allows oxygen to permeate the plasma. The oxygen concentration is increased and may oxygenate areas of previously blocked blood flow. The plasma can flow to areas where the red blood cells cannot go, and it reintroduces or reiterates perfusion in compromised tissue. This perfusion helps to create new capillaries and initiate cell growth for wound healing. Hyperbaric oxygen (HBO) is an excellent antibacterial agent aiding in the healing of infection by use of the oxygen free-radical enhancement. HBO stimulates the production of antioxidants called superoxide dismutase. HBO can heal certain wounds within as little as 10 to 20 treatments, without the use of medications or other methods.

Reviewing patient history information prior to initiating hyperbaric oxygen therapy

When vetting a patient for the initiation of hyperbaric oxygen therapy (HBOT), the patient's pertinent past medical history must be examined. Because of the effects of pressure and pure oxygen on the body's systems, the patient must be qualified to undergo pressure and oxygenation by checking the past medical history and testing questionable body systems. If the lungs have had previous trauma or disease, a pulmonary function test may be needed. If the heart has had disease or trauma in the past, an electrocardiogram or echocardiogram may be required. The hyperbaric physician needs to know if the patient smokes and how often. If the patient has a history of cancer and cancer medication, he or she may be contraindicated for HBOT. A retinal eye detachment, myopia, or cataracts is pertinent information for the hyperbaric physician. All body systems must be reviewed for potential complications before initiating HBOT.

Performing a utilization review of the patient

A utilization review is required of patients undergoing hyperbaric oxygen therapy. A utilization review is a hyperbaric physician's evaluation of whether or not the hyperbaric oxygen treatments are benefiting the patient, and if the course and type of hyperbaric treatments needs to be adjusted. The amount of hyperbaric treatment the patient receives before a utilization review is dependent on the diagnosis and indication for which that patient is being treated. Some patients will have a utilization review after 10 hyperbaric treatments, and other patients may have a utilization review after 20 or more treatments in the chamber. Factors to be considered during a utilization review are if the patient is tolerating the treatment, if the patient's wound is responding to the treatment, and if the partial pressure of oxygen values still justify the hyperbaric treatment. Other factors, such as the adequate control of infection and the presence of healthy, well-perfused, granulating tissue in the wound base, are also considered.

Verifying that the hyperbaric treatment is effective

The effectiveness of hyperbaric oxygen therapy (HBOT) on a particular patient may be evaluated, for example, through the use of a utilization review, a transcutaneous oxygen monitoring (TCOM) test, an X-ray, or a tissue culture. The patient's toleration of the hyperbaric oxygen treatment versus the potential benefit of the treatments must be taken into account when considering the effectiveness of hyperbaric oxygen therapy. If the patient has oxygen toxicity, intolerable confinement anxiety, or another medical illness, continued HBOT may not be in the patient's best interest. For example, the discontinuation of HBOT may need to be considered if TCOM test values are greater than 30 mmHg for a nondiabetic patient and greater than 40 mmHg for a diabetic patient. These values may mean that the wound is no longer hypoxic. These values may not be considered, however, if there is sufficient evidence that the condition of the patient or the response of the wound is due to HBOT.

Potential side effects evaluated during the course of treatment

The potential side effects of hyperbaric oxygen therapy (HBOT) must be considered and evaluated during the course of hyperbaric treatments. Barotrauma to the middle ear is a side effect of pressurization that is often considered. The risk for middle-ear barotrauma may be increased by anxiety, irritants such as smoking, unconsciousness, a language barrier, sedation, and intubation or tracheostomy. Cardiovascular conditions such as congestive heart failure (CHF), abnormal electrocardiogram, pacemaker, or defibrillator may be factors for consideration and may cause potential side effects such as a cardiac episode inside the hyperbaric chamber. Patients with CHF should be evaluated with an echocardiogram, and they must have an ejection fraction of greater than 30% before initiating HBOT. Oxygen toxicity is a rare side effect for patients inside a hyperbaric chamber, but it is a factor that needs great consideration because it can be serious.

Patient compliance factors that influence the treatment's overall effectiveness

The overall success of hyperbaric oxygen therapy (HBOT) is greatly affected by the patient's adherence to the plan of care, also known as treatment compliance. If the patient does not understand or does not comply with the hyperbaric facility rules or medical staff instructions, the effectiveness and safety of HBOT may be called into question. For example, if the patient continues to smoke during the course of the hyperbaric treatments, the ability of the oxygen to circulate freely in the bloodstream may be limited or restricted. If the patient is undergoing HBOT for a pressure ulcer, failure of the patient to offload the area or not to walk on that area may delay the effectiveness of HBOT. If the hyperbaric patient is diabetic and consumes foods that trigger a high blood glucose level, the ability of the wound to heal during hyperbaric oxygen therapy may be delayed.

Patient follow up after the hyperbaric treatment course concludes

Hyperbaric patient follow-up visits with the hyperbaric physician after the completion of the course of hyperbaric oxygen treatments may or may not be necessary. If the patient was diving for a nonhealing wound or ulcer and the wound has not been completely healed following a course of hyperbaric oxygen therapy, the patient may require follow-up visits for wound care and evaluation. Depending on the type of wound and severity of the ulcer, the patient may need one follow-up visit per week, or the patient may need up to three visits a week. The physician may decide that the patient only needs a home health nurse visit during the week. If the patient is diving for delayed radiation injuries, a follow-up visit with the hyperbaric physician is not typically necessary, but the patient may follow up with their own physician.

Additional therapies for post hyperbaric treatment

During and after the course of hyperbaric oxygen treatments, the patient may need additional therapies for their condition. The hyperbaric clinical staff should be aware of these therapies and should educate the patient on their options. For example, a transcutaneous oxygen test may determine if the patient needs to be revascularized, or even undergo an amputation. If the patient is receiving dialysis during the course of the hyperbaric treatments, the dialysis physician and the center need to be aware of the hyperbaric treatments and the potential side effects of receiving dialysis and hyperbaric therapies concurrently. A period of two to four hours may be needed in between dialysis and hyperbarics to prevent fluid onboarding and patient fatigue. The cardiac patient may need to be evaluated both during and after a course of hyperbaric treatments to prevent a cardiac episode. Communication between therapy medical centers and physicians is key to optimal patient health.

Responsibilities of a technologist during the posthyperbaric treatment visit

The hyperbaric technologist may be present during a part of the posthyperbaric follow-up visit to help evaluate the patient for barotrauma, vision changes, and other hyperbaric oxygen side effects. After a typical course of hyperbaric treatments (usually around 40 treatments), the technologist and the patient should have a solid rapport. The patient will be most comfortable with the hyperbaric technician, and the technologist should be able to facilitate communication between the hyperbaric physician and the patient regarding factors such as side effects and any other concerns. The technologist and the physician should work together to be sure that the patient is informed of any posthyperbaric concerns such as vision changes, wound care, and other health issues. For example, it is recommended that a patient wait at least six weeks after the last hyperbaric treatment before seeing an eye doctor.

Patient Care

Areas of education to cover during pretreatment briefing

The best outcome for patients undergoing hyperbaric oxygen therapy is achieved through patient and family education. Key areas to discuss before initiating hyperbaric oxygen therapy are as follows: what the patient should expect from the beginning of their treatments to the end, how the patient will be prepared for a chamber treatment, the risks and benefits of going under pressure, orientation to the department and the staff, the patient should be shown the chamber and how it works, the temperature changes that may occur for their body type, be informed of the noises present during a hyperbaric treatment, a staff member should demonstrate middle-ear equalization and then ask the patient to try it, potential confinement anxiety should be addressed, the patient should be aware of the potential for fire inside the hyperbaric chamber and how to prevent it, the patient should be completely informed before the consent is signed, and the patient should be aware of the facility's safety and policy procedures.

Potential side effects of exposure to hyperbaric doses of oxygen

During any hyperbaric oxygen treatment, there is a risk for oxygen toxicity. If the patient is being put at risk during a treatment or a procedure, he or she must be completely informed and consent must be given prior to any treatment. Some patients are more susceptible to oxygen toxicity than others, and each tissue reacts at different levels to oxygen toxicity. The two types of oxygen toxicity (central nervous system and pulmonary) represent two different groups of susceptible patients. Some manifestation of oxygen toxicity may even occur while breathing 100% oxygen at sea level. The hyperbaric patient is at risk for vision changes, chest tightness, difficulty breathing, ear ringing, twitching, sudden irritability, dizziness, nausea, hacking cough, seizures, lack of orientation, and loss of consciousness. The patient should understand that oxygen toxicity has a rare occurrence in hyperbaric oxygen therapy, but that there is a risk nonetheless.

Potential side effects related to changes in pressure

During any hyperbaric oxygen treatment, there is a risk for pressure-related injuries. If the patient is being put at risk during a procedure or treatment, he or she must be completely informed and consent must be given prior to the treatment. Any patient at any point during the course of their hyperbaric oxygen therapy (HBOT) may be susceptible to pressure-related injuries or side effects. Pressure-related injuries usually come in the form of barotrauma. Types of barotrauma are a pneumothorax (collapsed lung), middle-ear barotrauma, tooth squeeze, gastrointestinal aggravation, and sinus squeeze. A complete patient history will help to inform the hyperbaric staff of potential pressure-related injuries a particular patient could be susceptible to and how to prepare for their HBOT accordingly. It is important for the patient to be informed of possible pressure related injuries and side effects in order to help prevent them.

Medications that affect oxygen toxicity

Some medications, such as narcotics, steroids, anticonvulsants, and sedatives, may affect the potential for oxygen toxicity. A patient who is taking narcotics is more susceptible to oxygen toxicity because of the effect of a decrease in respiratory efforts. This leads to an increase in the partial pressures of carbon dioxide, which causes blood vessel dilation and an increase of oxygen diffusion. If a hyperbaric patient is taking a high dose of steroids, that patient's risk of oxygen toxicity becomes higher because of a high risk of seizure. The use of anticonvulsants during hyperbaric treatments may help to lessen or stop the seizure activity for oxygen toxicity. A hyperbaric patient may take a form of sedative to lessen the effects of confinement anxiety, but this medication may also be used to increase the seizure threshold for patients with a greater risk of oxygen toxicity.

Treating pneumothorax if it occurs during a hyperbaric treatment

A spontaneous pneumothorax is treated differently in a monoplace chamber versus in a multiplace chamber. Inside the multiplace chamber, an inside tender will treat a patient with a pneumothorax by inserting a chest tube to reduce the gas pressure in the lung. In the monoplace chamber, the patient must wait until the hyperbaric chamber is decompressed before he or she can receive proper treatment on the surface. Before chamber decompression, however, the chest tube tray must be in place, and the rapid response team must be standing by to rapidly insert the chest tube and treat the patient. If the patient has had a history of thoracic surgery, the procedure may have caused lesions to form, which may trap gas inside them. Patients may have had a history of lung disease, which may weaken the walls of the lung. These patients should receive chest X-rays prior to hyperbaric treatment, and if approved for HBOT, they must be compressed and decompressed slowly.

Informing the patient when they enter the compression and decompression stages

The pre-hyperbaric-therapy patient education and orientation process should inform the patient of the risks and side effects from the compression and decompression stages of the hyperbaric oxygen chamber. During the compression phase, the patient should be reminded to equalize or "clear" their ears. If the patient starts to experience pain in the ears during compression, he or she must know that they should communicate this as soon as possible to the hyperbaric tech. When the treatment at depth is completed, the patient should be informed that the chamber is going to decompress. During decompression, the patient will feel their ears equalizing automatically. If the patient has pain during decompression, it is called a "reverse squeeze." The patient should be aware of the side effects of decompression so as not to be alarmed when they happen.

Patients most at risk

Certain types of patients have a higher risk of oxygen toxicity than others, and they should be informed accordingly. Fever, increased carbon dioxide inhalation, hyperthyroidism, vitamin E deficiency, and history of epilepsy can contribute to increased seizure risk. Certain medications also increase the risk of seizure such as penicillin, steroids, epinephrine, a high dose of vitamin C, and narcotics. The likelihood of oxygen toxicity is lowered by decreasing the risks. A high fever may be reduced with medication prior to a hyperbaric oxygen treatment. The hyperbaric physician may instruct the patient to start a regimen of vitamin E. Other high-risk medications may be given at a lower dose or stopped completely.

Central nervous system oxygen toxicity vs. pulmonary oxygen toxicity

The two types of oxygen (O_2) toxicity are central nervous system (CNS), and pulmonary. CNS O_2 toxicity is short acting and mostly affects the brain, and pulmonary O_2 toxicity is long acting and mostly affects the lungs. The signs and symptoms of CNS O_2 toxicity can be remembered by the acronym VENTID-C, representing vision changes, ear ringing, nausea, tingling/twitching, irritability, dizziness, and convulsions. The signs and symptoms for pulmonary O_2 toxicity are as follows: chest tightness, a dry hacking cough, difficulty inhaling a full breath, and an increased rate and depth of respirations. Prevention of CNS O_2 toxicity includes having shorter and more frequent air breaks, and prevention of pulmonary O_2 toxicity includes having longer and less frequent air breaks.

How pulmonary oxygen toxicity is developed and subsequently treated

Pulmonary oxygen (O_2) toxicity is developed through the duration and exposure of high doses of O_2. It is rarely seen in clinical hyperbaric O_2 treatments because it mainly developed with the *U.S. Navy Diving Manual* treatment tables for decompression sickness. Exposure to pulmonary O_2 toxicity is measured in units called the unit pulmonary toxic dose (UPTD). 1 UPTD = 100% O_2 x 1 minute at 1 ATA. For example, at 30 fsw with 100% O_2, the UPTD is 71. The signs and symptoms of pulmonary O_2 toxicity are chest tightness, a dry hacking cough, difficulty inhaling a full breath, high respiratory rate, and abnormal depth of respirations. The air breaks for pulmonary O_2 toxicity should be longer and less frequent than with central nervous system O_2 toxicity.

Signs, symptoms, and management of hypoglycemia

Hypoglycemia is defined as low blood sugar. In this condition, the body's sugar count drops below normal levels. This can cause the patient to experience signs and symptoms such as excessive sweating, confusion, shakiness, trouble thinking or speaking clearly, and headaches. Hypoglycemia can be managed by eating meals at regular intervals and avoiding trigger foods (foods with a high sugar content). Patients who are typically hypoglycemic should have their blood glucose level checked prior to receiving treatment inside a hyperbaric chamber. A normal blood glucose level is 60 to 90 mg/dl. A mechanism of hyperbaric oxygen therapy typically drops the patient's glucose level by approximately 50 mg/dl. It is recommended that the diabetic or hypoglycemic patient's blood glucose level be at approximately 130 mg/dl before starting a hyperbaric treatment.

Differentiating between a hypoglycemic episode and oxygen toxicity symptoms

Hypoglycemia and oxygen toxicity both have similar signs and symptoms, and it may be difficult to differentiate between the two if the patient is inside a hyperbaric chamber. The technologist should keep in mind the distinctive signs and symptoms of hypoglycemia, such as excessive sweating, shakiness, headache, and confusion. Remember the acronym VENTID-C to distinguish for oxygen toxicity signs and symptoms: vision changes, ear ringing, nausea, tingling/twitching, irritability, dizziness, and convulsions. The patient inside a hyperbaric chamber may present with shakiness, confusion, or dizziness; all of these signs and symptoms could be attributed to either hypoglycemia or oxygen toxicity.

The best policy to follow is to give the patient an air break at once and call the hyperbaric physician. The treatment may need to be aborted in either case.

Methods for raising the patient's blood glucose level prior to a chamber treatment

Diabetic patients often become hypoglycemic when their blood glucose level drops below normal. To prevent this from happening inside the hyperbaric chamber, the patient should be told during the pretreatment education for hyperbaric oxygen therapy (HBOT) to eat meals at regular intervals and to take all medication as prescribed. The patient's blood glucose level should be checked prior to HBOT. The patient should be asked about the last time he or she ate and when the last dose of insulin was given. If the glucose level is found to be lower than 130 mg/dl, the patient should be given a nutritional supplement such as Glucerna or Ensure. Wait approximately 30 minutes before rechecking the glucose level. If the glucose level has not risen to an acceptable level or if it has dropped further, the hyperbaric physician may decide to cancel HBOT for that day.

Ways to prevent decompression sickness

Decompression sickness occurs when a body goes under pressure while breathing air and ascends from pressure faster than the body can compensate. During this process, the nitrogen in the air forms bubbles inside the bloodstream instead of dissolving into solution. These bubbles can form anywhere inside the body, and they may cause many symptoms or even death. The prevention of decompression sickness includes the following measures: decompression stops for the diver in the water or inside a recompression chamber, changing the diver's breathing gas mixture to include a higher dose of oxygen or other gases at specific times during the dive, and diving for shorter periods at depth.

Situations that predispose inside tenders to decompression sickness

There are several factors that may impact an inside tender's susceptibility to decompression sickness within a hyperbaric oxygen multiplace chamber. Predisposing scenarios include the following: the inside tender is pressurized to a treatment pressure of greater than 2 ATA, or 33 fsw, and he or she ascends from depth without decompressing adequately; the inside tender ascends to a height of greater than 18,000 feet right after a loss of aircraft pressurization; the inside tender takes a flight in an aircraft shortly after diving in water or inside a hyperbaric chamber; or the inside tender may have other risk factors such as dehydration, too much exertion at depth, or advanced age.

Decompression sickness vs. cerebral arterial gas embolism diagnosis

Cerebral arterial gas embolism (sometimes called air or gas embolism [AGE]) is a blood-flow obstruction in the form of gas bubbles circulating inside the arteries of the brain or heart. AGE can lead to certain death without immediate intervention. AGE is caused by not breathing properly upon ascent. Decompression sickness (DCS) is the formation of bubbles inside the bloodstream through the uptake and improper elimination of nitrogen. DCS can lead to severe pain and in some cases, even death. DCS is treated in a recompression chamber using the *U.S. Navy Diving Manual* treatment tables after a diver has experienced DCS signs and symptoms. AGE is treated in a recompression chamber if the diver resurfaces unconscious or if the diver goes unconscious within 10 minutes of resurfacing.

Pneumothorax

A pneumothorax is a collapsed lung that is caused by air or gas bubbles that may become trapped inside the pleural spaces in the lining of the lung. These gas bubbles can cause the lung to become detached from the chest wall, resulting in a deflated or collapsed lung. When a patient has a collapsed lung, it causes difficulty with breathing, and it may develop into a tension pneumothorax (when air enters the lung but does not leave it). A pneumothorax may be treated emergently by inserting a chest tube into the chest wall to relieve the pressure.

Potential risks associated with ascent from pressure

There are potential risks for the diver when ascending from pressure associated with the expansion of gas within the cavities of a human body. The middle-ear cavity is separated from the outside atmosphere by the eardrum. The middle ear requires equalization during compression, and it may even become painful on ascent from pressure, resulting in a reverse squeeze. The sinuses may contain a gas-filled cavity that is cut off from the outside by inflamed sinus membranes. Ascent from pressure may cause abdominal distension because of swallowed air or gases caused by digestion. The lungs themselves are a gas cavity that is relieved by breathing in and out normally. If the diver is not breathing during ascent, a pneumothorax or an arterial gas embolism may occur. Barodontalgia (*pressure + tooth + pain*) may occur when there is gas trapped inside the filling of a tooth.

Decreasing complications stemming from ascent from pressure

Some complications stemming from ascent from pressure may be decreased or relieved. During ascent, the gas space expands in the middle-ear cavity and causes a buildup of pressure against the eardrum, which is relieved by the "popping" of the eustachian tubes as they vent. The process may be facilitated by yawning and swallowing. The sinuses may become pressure blocked during ascent because of sinusitis, or inflammation of the sinus membranes. Taking nasal decongestants may help for the long term, but in the shorter interval, making a slow ascent is recommended. Abdominal distension may be relieved by burping or venting gas during ascent. Breathing normally will keep the lungs from becoming damaged and leading to a life-threatening event. There is not much a diver can do to relieve the pain of barodontalgia other than descend again. Regular dental checkups are recommended to prevent this complication.

Diagnoses that appear similar in nature to the classification of pulmonary barotrauma

Arterial gas embolism, pneumothorax, tension pneumothorax, subcutaneous emphysema, and mediastinal emphysema are all similar conditions that may be related to pulmonary barotrauma. An arterial gas embolism is when gas bubbles enter the arterial circulation and block blood flow. It is caused by retaining air in the lungs upon ascent. A pneumothorax is when air is trapped between the chest wall and the lung in the pleural space. When the lung retains the air pressure, it is called a tension pneumothorax. These two may be caused by lung disease or trauma. Mediastinal emphysema happens when the gas in the lung is forced through the tissue into the mediastinal tissues; when the gas migrates to the neck, it is called subcutaneous emphysema. These emphysemas may be caused by overinflation of the lungs in diving exercises and are called pulmonary overinflation syndromes.

Treating each type of emphysema as related to pulmonary barotrauma

The two types of emphysema are mediastinal and subcutaneous. Mediastinal symptoms include pain near or under the breastbone, chest tightness, and pain radiating to the shoulder and back that is increased upon inhalation. The symptoms for subcutaneous emphysema include a "full" feeling in the neck, an obvious bulge in the neck area, and a crackling sound upon adding pressure to the neck. The treatment for both mediastinal and subcutaneous emphysema are the same and include breathing 100% oxygen at the surface. For more severe symptoms, a shallow recompression of the diver in a hyperbaric chamber is recommended.

Treating each type of pneumothorax as related to pulmonary barotrauma

When the lung tissues are torn and air is allowed to become trapped in the pleural space between the chest wall and lung, it is called a pneumothorax. This condition may be improved by the reabsorption of 100% oxygen into the lung, or in severe cases, a chest tube may need to be inserted. When the damaged lung allows air to be inhaled, but not exhaled, it causes a buildup of pressure and is called a tension pneumothorax. This condition is treated with a chest tube and recompression of the diver in a hyperbaric chamber.

Treating cerebral arterial gas embolism as related to pulmonary barotrauma

An arterial gas embolism (AGE) is caused by an overinflation of the lungs that obstructs blood flow in the arteries of the brain and heart. The symptom that is often the first noted is unconsciousness within 10 minutes of a diver surfacing. Other symptoms may include paralysis, numbness, weakness, vertigo, convulsions, nausea, vomiting, hearing and vision changes, and tremors. An AGE may be aggravated by other pulmonary overinflation syndromes such as mediastinal and subcutaneous emphysema, or a pneumothorax. An AGE may be treated with first aid, 100% oxygen on the surface, and immediate recompression in a hyperbaric chamber.

Cardiopulmonary complications that could arise during hyperbaric treatment

Cardiopulmonary symptoms, or "the chokes" may occur due to the circulation of the lungs becoming congested. The chokes is caused by profuse intravascular bubbling due to decompression sickness. Chest pain that is made worse by inspiration of air into the lungs and aggravated by coughing is a symptom of the chokes. Hyperventilation may also occur. Increasing lung congestion may lead to circulatory collapse, loss of consciousness, and death. Recompression of the patient must be started immediately. Carefully observe the patient for signs of a pneumothorax if shortness of breath is present. Do not recompress the patient if a pneumothorax is the only symptom. If there are other signs and symptoms of decompression sickness or air gas embolism present, recompression is indicated, even with a known pneumothorax.

Signs and symptoms of severe cardiovascular distress

Cardiovascular distress can occur from different conditions — all related to failure of the heart pump to maintain the pressure needed to circulate enough blood for the body's needs. The most noted symptom of cardiovascular distress is shortness of breath that may worsen with exercise, or even laying down. Edema of the legs and excessive tiredness are also notable symptoms. Other symptoms could present such as a high heart rate or palpitations, nausea and lack of appetite, difficulty thinking or confusion, chronic coughing, and differing degrees of chest pain or pressure.

Responding to a patient experiencing cardiovascular distress in a multiplace chamber

If a patient is experiencing cardiovascular distress inside of a multiplace hyperbaric chamber, the inside tender must notify the chamber operator immediately and perform basic life support as needed. The chamber operator in turn must notify the hyperbaric physician and nurse and must call for a rapid response team to be on hand. The hyperbaric physician must direct the actions of the inside tender, and if necessary, extra personnel must be locked in the chamber as soon as possible to perform life-saving techniques such as pushing drugs and fluids that the inside tender may not be qualified to perform. The use of a defibrillator inside the hyperbaric chamber is prohibited. The hyperbaric chamber should not be decompressed until the hyperbaric physician directs.

Responding to a patient experiencing cardiovascular distress in a monoplace chamber

If a patient is experiencing cardiovascular distress inside of a monoplace hyperbaric chamber, the chamber operator must stop travel immediately, and notify the hyperbaric physician and nurse. A rapid response team should also be notified and should be standing by to treat the patient as soon as the chamber surfaces and the patient is moved to a nonhyperbaric stretcher and all linens are removed. The reason for this is if the patient requires defibrillation, the oxygen-saturated mattress and linens may catch fire. The hyperbaric chamber must not be decompressed until the patient is breathing, or unless the technologist is directed otherwise by the hyperbaric physician.

Known risks and approval process for pacemakers and defibrillators

Internal pacemakers and defibrillators may be approved for use in a hyperbaric oxygen chamber, only with on-hand documentation of approval from the manufacturer. The reasons for the contraindication of pacemakers and defibrillators are a potential for malfunction when pressurized, and if the device is activated, there is a risk of fire and explosion inside the hyperbaric chamber. To obtain the manufacturer's recommendations concerning the pressurization of these devices, you must first obtain some information from the patient. The patient will typically carry a device identification card, which will have all the information required to contact the manufacturer for approval. If this is not the case, obtain the patient's social security number and start contacting popular device manufacturers until success is achieved.

Universally recognized infection control policies

Standard precautions for infection control are generally recognized throughout hospital systems and adopted as policy. Hand hygiene is required by the policies provided by the Centers for Disease Control or the World Health Organization for healthcare settings. Hand hygiene should be performed before and after every patient contact. In a wound care setting, gloves are used for dressing changes, wound measurement, and blood draws. Gloves, gowns, and face shields are used for irrigation and debridement. Sharps such as needles should be disposed of in a sharps container. Needles should not be recapped. Exam chairs, stretchers, wheelchairs, and ancillary equipment should be disinfected using approved cleaners. Soiled linens should be disposed of properly and in a timely manner. Biohazard bags should be used as necessary.

Typical circumstances that call for disinfecting the chamber between patient use

Under normal conditions, the hyperbaric oxygen chambers should be cleaned and disinfected with approved cleaners once a week during the weekly preventative maintenance. If the hyperbaric patient is known to have an infectious disease such as MRSA, *Clostridium difficile*, etc., then the chamber must be cleaned and disinfected before the next patient's treatment. After the chamber is cleaned, it must be compressed to idle pressure without a patient inside to vent the fumes. The hyperbaric chamber should also be cleaned prior to the next patient's treatment if there is any residue inside the chamber left from the previous patient.

Cross-contamination impact to the patient, medical staff, and equipment

The hyperbaric and wound care staff should be ever vigilant to ensure the prevention of cross-contamination of infectious diseases between patients. The cleansing and disinfecting of all surfaces in the clinic is critical to the prevention of cross-contamination. Not only are the patients at risk of sharing infection, but the wound care and hyperbaric staff are also at risk. Great care should be taken to prevent the sharing of topical medications, wound cleansers, gauze pads, and other supplies and equipment. Equipment such as blood pressure cuffs and oxygen saturation leads should be disinfected between use.

Reasons that some patients are reluctant to undergo hyperbaric treatment

Patients may be reluctant to undergo hyperbaric oxygen (HBO) treatments for a variety of reasons. The most popular reason for treatment reluctance is confinement anxiety, or claustrophobia. To put the patient at ease, a tour of the facility and a chamber treatment demonstration during the hyperbaric orientation process may be helpful. Another reason for treatment reluctance is cultural superstitions. Certain cultures may see the hyperbaric chamber as taboo. Education to the patient and the patient's family may help with this issue. Another example of reluctance is that the patient may not believe in the science behind HBO theory. Patient success stories and HBO literature may be offered to the patient in this situation.

Facilitating patient comfort during the treatment

Patient comfort inside the hyperbaric oxygen chamber is of utmost importance for their continued compliance with the treatment course. If the patient is continually too hot or too cold inside the hyperbaric chamber, he or she may not wish to continue undergoing treatments. The hyperbaric technologist should ask the patient beforehand if their body tends to run hot or cold. Be sure the cooler temperatured patient has plenty of blankets available to them. The patient who is usually warmer temperatured may be informed to take off blankets if they become warm. The technologist may also compress the warm patient at a slower rate to prevent overheating. There is no air-conditioning system inside the monoplace chamber. The system that the hyperbaric technologist may control to facilitate patient comfort is the proper use of the compression valve and the plateau ventilation valve. During compression, the valve may be opened or closed to increase or decrease airflow. After compression is achieved, this function is transferred to the plateau valve.

General patient comfort techniques

When a patient is uncomfortable during a hyperbaric treatment, there are steps the hyperbaric technologist may take in order to calm the patient. The communications system allows the Technologist to speak with the patient. Ask the patient to breathe normally. If the patient is too hot, tell him or her to remove blankets or clothing. The technologist may turn up the air flow with the compression valve or the plateau valve. This action will only increase the airflow, not lower the temperature. If the patient is known to become hot inside the chamber, take the patient down to pressure at a slower than normal rate. If the patient cannot tolerate the treatment, the technologist may abort the dive, but explain to the patient that the chamber door will not open until the pressure equalizes, which takes 10 to 15 minutes depending on the treatment depth. When aborting the dive for anxiety, call the physician and give aid as needed.

Assisting a patient in overcoming claustrophobia/confinement anxiety

Claustrophobia/confinement anxiety can be a significant hurdle for hyperbaric patients to overcome. Multiplace chambers may lessen anxiety with the presence of a tender. Otherwise, any chamber with accessibility to television or radio and the ability to communicate via intercom can provide some comfort to the patient. The medical director may also prescribe a daily antianxiety medication for the course of hyperbaric oxygen therapy (HBOT). The optimal way to reduce initial apprehension is thorough patient education. Aside from a facility tour and hyperbaric staff introductions, a complete HBOT orientation should review what the patient should expect from the minute he or she arrives at the center until his or her departure each day, the type of commitment that is required to fully complete the course of treatments, and which items are prohibited and why. Lastly, assert that the patient may decide to exit the chamber at any time. Taking these steps will help to build the patient's confidence in the hyperbaric therapy process.

Hyperbaric technologist's role in wound care

The hyperbaric technologist may be required to assist in the wound care of patients under the supervision of the hyperbaric registered nurse. On-the-job training will be provided, if necessary, for wound care techniques. If desired, the hyperbaric technologist may seek wound care certification as part of his or her continued education. The hyperbaric technologist may learn to perform wound dressing changes, negative pressure therapy, compression wraps, and other techniques as part of the complete hyperbaric therapy process. The technologist must learn infection control and wound cleansing techniques as part of the foundation of basic wound care.

Basic wound care principles

The hyperbaric technologist must learn and be aware of the principles and technologies that will lead to optimal wound healing. Infection control of the wound is a critical part of the healing process. If the patient has had a long-standing wound, the area around the wound is more likely to acquire bacteria and subsequent infection. The presence of peripheral artery disease (PAD) must be assessed in patients with areas of ischemia. A transcutaneous oximetry test will help determine the patient's viability for hyperbaric oxygen therapy and the extent of PAD. Proper wound cleansing and irrigation are critical to the removal of bacteria, surface debris, and the reduction of inflammation. Wound debridement is the removal of necrotic bone and tissue. Oral antibiotics will help to disinfect the wound area. The final part of the process is the application of topical antimicrobial medications and dressing the wound.

Common wound types

The hyperbaric technologist should be familiar with common wound types and their basic treatments. Wound classifications and stages are helpful to know when categorizing wounds for specific wound treatment regimens. Pressure ulcers may develop when a patient is confined to a wheelchair or a bed. Off-loading the pressure wound is critical to healing pressure ulcers. Venous ulcers occur in the lower legs and are the most common type of ulcer. Venous ulcers develop from pressure inside the veins of the legs. Diabetic ulcers typically develop from poor diet and glucose control, which may result in neuropathy of the extremities. Surgical wounds may be compromised by underlying factors such as infection. Arterial ulcers occur due to blood vessel blockage. All of these wound types may become necrotic or infected, or they may become compromised by other medical conditions.

Examples of wound dressings and topical medications that are frequently used

The hyperbaric and wound care physician may order multiple medications (topical and oral) and wound dressings for patients in the wound care program. It is the technologist's responsibility to be familiar with these products. The types of dressings include the following: antimicrobial, alginate, biosynthetic, collagen, composite, compression, foam, gauze, multilayered systems, conforming wraps, contact layers, hydrogel, hydrocolloid, and transparent film dressings. The types of cleansers include the following: saline, skin cleanser, and wound cleanser. Creams and oils may be used to keep the skin from getting dry under the dressings. Enzymes or debriding agents may ordered by the physician for daily application. Device therapy such as vacuum-assisted closure or hyperbaric oxygen therapy may be ordered.

Debridement

If necrotic tissue or bone is present in the wound bed, a procedure called debridement may be necessary to further the wound healing process. This can only be performed by a doctor. Classification and wound staging may not be accomplished until the wound has been debrided. Debridement is necessary to prevent infection because necrotic tissue is a medium for pathogens. Types of debridement include the following: surgical, sharp, conservative sharp, ultrasonic, mechanical, enzymatic, and autolytic. Debridement selection factors are based on the extent of necrotic tissue, pain, infection, vascular status, coagulation status, and facility policy.

Nurse and technologist required documents

Documentation is an important part of the wound healing process. Proper documentation enables the medical staff to keep track of the patient's wound progress and to develop a plan of care. The hyperbaric technologist must document all elements of the safety program including safety checklists and preventative maintenance schedules. For each patient and each dive, the technologist must complete a dive profile, usually on a treatment record document. The patient's vital signs may also be recorded on this document. The hyperbaric nurse must complete plan-of-care documents on each patient and record information from physician visits including physician orders, pharmaceutical, and supplemental treatment notes.

Transcutaneous Oxygen (tcpO2) Technology

Transcutaneous oxygen technology

Transcutaneous oxygen monitoring is used to determine the amount and quality of the partial pressure of oxygen circulating in the bloodstream in a certain area of the body. This is accomplished by attaching noninvasive heated electrodes to the indicated parts of the body where blood flow is questionable. The partial pressure of oxygen is measured in millimeters of mercury (mmHg). The electrodes are heated to 45° Celsius and calibrated while attached to the monitor at 160 mmHg (plus or minus 5 mmHg). At sea level, the amount of oxygen inspired is translated to 160 mmHg on a patient without vascular disease; whereas at the arterial level, the amount of oxygen is at 100 mmHg; and at the cellular level, the amount of oxygen is 60 mmHg. The electrodes will detect the amount of oxygen at the cellular level: 60 mmHg for normal vascularization. The electrodes are attached to the skin for 15 minutes. At the end of the time interval, the baseline readings are taken. A reading below 40 mmHg indicates hypoxia. The value increases to greater than 100 mmHg in a normally vascularized patient during the oxygen challenge, in which the patient breathes 100% oxygen on a nonrebreather mask for 10 minutes. These values are translated onto a medical document for physician interpretation.

Principles of transcutaneous oximetry and how to interpret the measurements

The transcutaneous oxygen monitor detects hypoxia. Wound healing is impaired with hypoxia or decreasing partial pressures of oxygen ($tcPO_2$). A $tcPO_2$ reading of less than 40 mmHg is associated with impaired wound healing. The $tcPO_2$ test measures oxygen molecules, not saturation. Electrodes are attached to a fixation ring on the skin. The electrodes are heated to 44 to 45° Celsius to cause local dilation of pores and local dilation of capillaries and to make the hemoglobin release oxygen more readily. This allows the oxygen to permeate through the epidermis under the electrode head. Normal sea-level $tcPO_2$ values on room air are as follows: average calf, 60 mmHg; average foot, 56 mmHg. Sea-level $tcPO_2$ values on 100% oxygen are as follows: average calf, 204 mmHg; average foot, 170 mmHg. In normal patients, breathing oxygen always increases $ctPO_2$ to greater than 100 mmHg. $tcPO_2$ values on the calf are always higher than those on the foot.

Typical patient response to transcutaneous oximetry

The patient's response to transcutaneous oxygen ($tcPO_2$) may be indicative of a possible therapeutic response to hyperbaric oxygen therapy (HBOT). For example, a diabetic patient with a high enough $tcPO_2$ during the oxygen challenge for a diabetic foot ulcer has high expectation of a therapeutic response in the hyperbaric chamber. On the other hand, the same patient with a decrease in $tcPO_2$ is predictive of failure to respond to HBOT. A patient response to elevation of the lower extremity during the $tcPO_2$ while breathing air at 1ATA may reveal hemodynamically significant peripheral vascular disease in the case of a low baseline measurement. Any decrease from the baseline of 20% or more is considered to be significant. The lower that the $tcPO_2$ value below 40 mmHg is, the more severe the hypoxia and failure of wound healing will be. Room-air $tcPO_2$ measurement is a good way to determine if a patient will benefit from either revascularization or hyperbaric oxygen therapy, or both.

Applications of transcutaneous oximetry

There are several applications for transcutaneous oxygen testing, such as evaluation of peripheral arterial occlusive disease or the initial selection of patients for treatment modalities. Transcutaneous oxygen monitoring can be used preoperatively to assess postsurgical wound healing failure risk in selected patients. Assessment of transcutaneous oxygen ($tcPO_2$) may be done following peripheral arterial angioplasty and/or revascularization and following edema reduction and control. It can also be used during adjunctive hyperbaric oxygen treatments and periodically for reassessment. A baseline room-air $tcPO_2$ study can be used to define the presence or absence of clinically significant hypoxia on all diabetic wounds and on all lower extremity wounds based on abnormal physician exam results.

Transcutaneous Oxygen Monitors and Related Equipment

Various transcutaneous oxygen monitors and related equipment

The various transcutaneous oxygen monitor types for room air and hyperbaric use are the Tina Radiometer 400 series (six-lead monitor), and the Perimed PeriFlux System 5000. The PeriFlux System is a four-lead monitor, but a second monitor can be connected with cables and software for an eight-lead oximetry test. Variations on the PeriFlux system include a laser Doppler probe, one or two heat sensors, a combined transcutaneous oxygen and transcutaneous carbon dioxide test function; and the ability to measure toe pressure, skin perfusion, and pulse volume.

Operating functions of a transcutaneous oxygen monitor

The functions of the transcutaneous oxygen monitor are time, high alarm, low alarm, temperature in Celsius, and partial pressure of oxygen (PO_2) in mmHg. The timer is used to shut off the heating element when the time runs out. The timer is adjustable up to 8 hours in increments of 30 minutes. The high alarm is set to sound when the high value is reached. The high alarm is adjustable up to 2000 in increments of 1 mmHg. The low alarm is set to sound when the low value is reached, and it is adjustable down to zero from 2000 in increments of 1 mmHg. The temperature setting affects the heating element of the electrode, and it may be adjusted from 37 to 45° Celsius in increments of 0.5°. The PO_2 setting detects the actual PO_2 in the room and may be adjustable from zero to 2000 in 1-mmHg increments.

How to calibrate and verify calibration of the transcutaneous oxygen monitor

The transcutaneous oxygen monitor must be calibrated before use on a patient. When the monitor is switched on, the electrodes must be placed into the calibration sockets. The display will show "C" or a "CAL" depending on the type of monitor. Push the CAL button for each electrode. A flashing light will signal that the electrode is calibrating. During calibration, the electrode heats up to 45° Celsius. The partial pressure of oxygen values will appear on the display. At this time, the monitor will perform internal checks, and it will fix the high and low calibration points. The calibration will take from 5 to 10 minutes. Once the calibration is complete, the monitor will beep and the flashing light will become steady. While in the calibration socket, the electrode is detecting the amount of oxygen in the air, reading as 160 mmHg plus or minus 5 mmHg. Wait at least one minute before attaching electrodes to the patient so as to watch for "drift." If drift occurs beyond plus or minus 5 mmHg, recalibrate the electrode.

Sensor electrode and the parts of the transcutaneous oxygen monitor

Core components of the transcutaneous oxygen monitor (TCOM) are as follows: the monitor (there are many models and types), electrode cables, power adapter, and a computer cable (in some models). The TCOM may operate on battery power. The battery charges when the power adapter is plugged in. The electrode cable is attached to the back or the side of the monitor, depending on the type. The electrode head is placed into the calibration socket. The computer cable may be attached to the computer in order to produce a printed TCOM report (in certain models). The electrode head consists of a heating element and sensor, a gas permeable membrane, and the electrolyte solution. The electrode heating element causes local dilation of the pores and capillaries, and it causes hemoglobin to release oxygen more readily. The sensor measures the amount of energy in the electrolyte solution. The $tcPO_2$ monitor translates this amount into mmHg of PO_2 based on the PO_2 calibration setting.

Membrane care and replacement of the transcutaneous oxygen monitor leads

The manufacturer Radiometer recommends changing the electrode membranes every two weeks. This membrane change must be documented in a membrane maintenance binder. Membraning kits must be kept on hand at the hyperbaric facility. The membraning kit contains a membrane removal tool, polishing cloths, electrolyte solution, and 12 membrane cartridges. The procedure to change the membranes begins with using the membrane removal tool to remove the elastic bands around the electrode head. Next, peel off the old membrane (this may be done by rubbing a gloved finger over the electrode head). Dry off the old electrolyte solution and use the round cloth to polish the electrode head to remove any particles. Carefully place three drops of electrolyte solution onto the electrode head. Turn the electrode head upside down, and press down onto the new membrane cartridge, applying slow, steady pressure. Carefully check the new membrane for bubbles in the electrolyte. Redo the membraning process if bubbles appear.

Transcutaneous oxygen monitor care

Cleaning and disinfecting the transcutaneous oxygen monitor (TCOM) should take place after every patient test. To clean the probes, mix a solution of mild detergent and water and use a lint-free cloth to wipe down the monitor and the leads and sensors. Isopropyl alcohol 70% may also be used to disinfect the TCOM. The sensor/probe connectors should never be immersed in any type of solution. Do not use strong solvents such as acetone, benzene, or chloroform to clean the monitor or the probes. Any blood or dirt should be removed from the leads and sensors as soon as possible.

Methods of troubleshooting the transcutaneous oxygen monitor

There are a few general methods for troubleshooting a transcutaneous oxygen monitor. If the monitor fails to start, wait two minutes and try again. Be sure to check the power supply cables and the fuses. For an atypical value from a sensor, recalibrate the probe. Check that the probe is clean and the membrane is free of bubbles. Ensure the probe/sensor has been attached to the skin correctly, and check for air leaks around the attached probe by passing oxygen over the site while watching for a rise in value. If an error message is displayed on the unit, record the error, and look it up in the user manual.

Transcutaneous Oxygen Testing Procedure

How to select sites for the transcutaneous oxygen monitoring leads

Site selection for the transcutaneous oxygen monitoring (TCOM) leads is an important step in the TCOM testing process. Typically, the physician and the hyperbaric technologist collaborate on lead placement. A perfect site for lead placement is a flat surface, free of hair (use a razor), that is approximately one inch in diameter. Sites to be avoided include the following: any sharply curved part of the anatomy, an area of draining from a wound, the wound itself, a major blood vessel (pulse site), the plantar surface of the foot, a callous, a bony prominence (such as the malleolus, where there are very few capillaries present), and wrinkles on the skin (if there is no other option, smooth the wrinkles out while applying the fixation ring). Standardized sites may be used for consistency. For example, two leads at the transmetatarsal amputation level and two leads at the below-knee amputation level. These are preselected based on blood vessel anatomy and typical amputation levels. Nonstandard sites may be proximal and distal to the wound, and also the tissue surrounding the wound may be considered.

Preparing the site for the transcutaneous oxygen monitor leads

Site preparation is the most important step in the transcutaneous oxygen test. If the site is not prepared correctly, oxygen may leak from the room air into the electrolyte solution. Site-preparation supplies include the following: a razor, alcohol wipes, tape, fixation rings, and contact liquid (electrolyte solution). Remove any barriers from the skin. Shave all hair that is present at the site. Hair under the fixation ring will cause room air to leak into the electrode, giving a false-high reading. Clean the skin by removing dirt and oil with the alcohol wipes. Soap and water may be needed if thick ointments are present. Remove any loose skin by "stripping" with the tape. Apply the fixation ring securely to the skin. Tape may be used to ensure there is no leak. Place three to four drops of contact solution into the fixation ring. Finally, place the electrode lead into the fixation ring by tightening it a quarter turn clockwise, and then secure the cable to the patient with tape. As a precaution, do not place tape over the electrode head because this will compress it into the skin and may restrict circulation.

Common interpretation methods for the transcutaneous oxygen test

The transcutaneous oxygen test is for the evaluation of nonhealing wounds. Normal values of partial pressure of oxygen ($tcPO_2$) skin measurements range between 50 and 70 mmHg. A $tcPO_2$ value of less than 40 mmHg (less than 50 mmHg in diabetic patients) represents a hypoxic wound. The leg elevation portion of the test may indicate lower leg peripheral arterial occlusive disease. After revascularization, if the value raises greater than 30 mmHg, the wound has a significant chance of healing. The presence of inflammation and edema at the measurement site may obstruct a true value. A value of less than 100 mmHg in a hyperbaric chamber may indicate no benefit of hyperbaric oxygen therapy to the patient. The regional perfusion index will help determine if a low $tcPO_2$ value is a local or a central issue.

Reference site for the transcutaneous oxygen monitor

The reference site, or control site, may be used to obtain a normal reading in an area of good perfusion, typically close to the central circulation. The patient's chest at the left second intercostal space is the usual reference site unless there is an interruption of normal blood flow to that area. The regional perfusion index (RPI) is a calculation of a distal value PO_2 (typically on the foot) divided by the reference-site PO_2. For example, the baseline foot PO_2 value is 40, and the reference site PO_2 is 80. The equation would read 40/80 = 0.5. The RPI is 0.5. The RPI is beneficial in determining if a low partial pressure of oxygen reading is a local or a central circulation problem (arterial hypoxemia).

Room-air and in-chamber transcutaneous oxygen monitoring

A normobaric, or room-air transcutaneous oxygen monitoring (TCOM) is a partial pressure of oxygen ($tcPO_2$) test in which baseline and leg elevation on room air testing and an oxygen challenge with 100% oxygen are performed. A hyperbaric or in-chamber TCOM is a $tcPO_2$ test performed inside the hyperbaric chamber. A baseline is completed outside the chamber on room air. The patient is then pressurized to 2 atmospheres absolute (ATA) or 14.7 psig. After recording the values, the patient is further pressurized to 2.5 ATA or 29.4 psig, and then the final values are recorded. The normal values for an in-chamber TCOM are 700 mmHg at 2 ATA and 800 mmHg at 2.5 ATA for the leg, and 500 mmHg at 2 ATA and 600 mmHg at 2.5 ATA for the foot. However, the probability of success or failure of diabetic lower extremity ulcers is a $tcPO_2$ of greater than 200 mmHg. This $tcPO_2$ has a 75% positive predictive value of a successful hyperbaric oxygen therapy outcome.

Documentation and data recording procedure for transcutaneous oxygen monitoring

The data recording procedure for transcutaneous oxygen monitoring (TCOM) starts with calibration. After switching the monitor on, attach the electrode leads to the calibration sockets, and push "CAL." At this point, the fixation rings may be attached to the patient, and the placement may be documented on the TCOM test sheet. After calibration is complete, attach the leads to the patient. Press "start" to begin the TCOM test. First, the monitor will collect the baseline values after 15 minutes. Record the baseline values in conjunction with the lead placement on the TCOM test sheet. The next 15 minutes is the segment during which the patient's legs are elevated. Record these values on the test sheet. After this, the patient's legs are lowered back to normal level for five minutes to give the values time to get back to the baseline. Record these values as well. Last is the oxygen challenge during which the patient is given 100% oxygen via a nonrebreather mask. After the oxygen challenge values are recorded, the test is complete, and the TCOM test sheet is ready for physician interpretation.

Practice Test

Practice Questions

1. Which of the gas laws states the following: "Solubility of a gas in a liquid is directly proportional to the pressure of the gas?"
   a. Henry's
   b. Boyle's
   c. Charles'
   d. Dalton's

2. An air tank contains 0.2 moles of oxygen and 0.3 moles of nitrogen. The tank is in standard pressure (1 atm) and temperature. What is the partial pressure of the nitrogen?
   a. 0.3 atm
   b. 0.5 atm
   c. 0.6 atm
   d. 0.8 atm

3. A person inhales at a pressure of 3 atm, filling his lungs with 0.9 L of gas. The person moves to a pressure of 101.32 kPa, without a change in temperature, and without exhaling. What is the volume of the gas at this new pressure?
   a. 0.3 L
   b. 0.6 L
   c. 1.8 L
   d. 2.7 L

4. The abbreviation ATA is used to signify which of the following pressures?
   a. Atmospheric pressure
   b. Gauge pressure
   c. Absolute pressure
   d. Partial pressure

5. Which of the gas laws states the following: "Total pressure exerted by the mixture of nonreactive gases is equal to the sum of the partial pressures of individual gases?"
   a. Dalton's Law
   b. Henry's Law
   c. Boyle's Law
   d. Charles' Law

6. What is function of the respiratory system?
   a. To deliver carbon dioxide to body tissues
   b. To exchange respiratory gases between blood and air
   c. To remove carbon monoxide generated by cellular respiration
   d. To remove oxygen from the body

7. Which of the following is a characteristic of the cardiovascular system?
   a. Veins carry blood away from the heart
   b. Arteries, veins, and capillaries are three blood vessel types that connect directly to the heart.
   c. Arteries become progressively smaller as they leave the heart
   d. The walls of veins are much thicker than the walls of arteries

8. When the blood level of carbon dioxide increases above normal, your brain___________
   a. increases the rate and depth of respiration.
   b. decreases the rate and increases the depth of respiration.
   c. decreases the rate and depth of respiration.
   d. increases the rate and decreases the depth of respiration.

9. Which of the following conditions increase the likelihood of CNS oxygen toxicity?
   a. Hyperthermia
   b. Vitamin A deficiency
   c. Hypothyroidism
   d. All the above

10. Barotrauma can occur during SCUBA diving because of______________
   a. ascending while exhaling.
   b. inhaling while diving from 100 to 150 feet.
   c. failure to equalize middle ear pressure.
   d. none of the above.

11. Which of the following is most likely associated with a form of decompression sickness called the "staggers?"
   a. Gas bubbles in pulmonary artery
   b. Ringing in the ears
   c. Purple skin rash
   d. All the above

12. Hypothermia is a medical emergency and is characterized with which of the following?
   a. Body loses heat slower than it can produce heat
   b. Decreased body temperature interferes with metabolism and enzyme function
   c. Occurs when your body temperature is above 95°F
   d. Low body temperature causes heat stroke

13. Which of the following is a symptom of acute embolism?
   a. Hearing loss
   b. Tissue death
   c. Blood clotting
   d. Osteonecrosis

14. What mechanism is responsible for nitrogen narcosis during a deep sea dive?
   a. Increased pressure causes nitrogen to dissolve into body tissues
   b. Breathing pressurized oxygen pushes nitrogen out of tissue
   c. High pressure causes nitrogen bubbles to enter bloodstream
   d. Decreased pressure causes blood to exchange oxygen to nitrogen

15. Which of the following does NOT increase the risk of decompression sickness?
    a. High body fat
    b. Dehydration
    c. Diving in warm water
    d. Drinking alcohol

16. Hyperbaric oxygen therapy (HBOT) is approved for the following conditions EXCEPT:
    a. Arthritis
    b. Arterial gas embolism
    c. Delayed radiation injury
    d. Anemia

17. Transcutaneous oxygen monitoring is used for which of the following?
    a. To measure tissue hypoxia around problem wounds
    b. To determine patient's need for transcutaneous oxygen tension
    c. To prevent tissue death
    d. All the above

18. Which of the following is a potential side effect of HBOT?
    a. Seizure
    b. Organ damage
    c. Temporary myopia
    d. All the above

19. HBOT is a beneficial treatment for arterial gas embolism due to what mechanism?
    a. Gases are released faster from the tissue than the rate they are degassed from the body
    b. Nitrogen is removed from the arteries and carried only in the veins until removed from the body
    c. Nitrogen bubbles located in body tissues and blood vessels are reduced in their size
    d. All of the above

20. You are monitoring a patient who is at the latter stages of HBOT in a multiperson chamber. You notice the patient beginning to show twitching around the mouth during the therapy. What is your immediate action?
    a. Take patient's vital signs
    b. Immediately decompress the chamber
    c. Take patient off oxygen
    d. Perform a neurological examination

21. Your patient has a nonhealing wound in his leg. Which of the following hyperbaric oxygen therapy protocols would you use for treating this condition?
    a. 30 minutes 50% oxygen at 1 ATA twice a day
    b. 0.5 hour 100% oxygen at 2 ATA once a day
    c. 60 minutes 50% oxygen at 1 ATA once a day
    d. 1.5 hour 100% oxygen at 2 ATA twice a day

22. Which of the following mechanisms is NOT a beneficial effect of HBOT for the treatment of osteoradionecrosis?
a. Promotes blood vessel formation
b. Induces osteoclast bone cell formation
c. Promotes connective tissue formation
d. Decreases tissue hypoxia

23. When treatment is delayed for more than 6 hours, HBOT for decompression sickness should include recompression to________________ with 50-50 mixture of nitrox or heliox breathing gases.
a. 60 feet for 260 minutes
b. 60 feet for 50 minutes
c. 165 feet for 30 minutes
d. 165 feet for 285 minutes

24. You are treating a patient who has finished a 20-meter, 30-minute SCUBA diving trip an hour ago. The patient is showing the following signs: breathing difficulties, upper back pain, bruising of the eyelids, and hearing difficulties. Which of the following is the most likely cause for all of these symptoms?
a. Arterial gas embolism
b. Barotrauma
c. Carbon monoxide poisoning
d. Nitrogen narcosis

25. Which of the following is a characteristic of transcutaneous oxygen monitoring?
a. Transcutaneous oxygen monitoring measures tissue oxygen levels from inside the skin.
b. Transcutaneous oxygen monitoring was originally developed to measure oxygen content in diabetic patients.
c. Transcutaneous oximetry cannot be used with newborns.
d. Transcutaneous oximetry measures blood oxygen content without invading the skin.

26. Complete the following sentence: Low tissue oxygen concentration______________
a. increases the likelihood of tissue death.
b. is a symptom of oxygen toxicity.
c. can be treated with high-altitude therapy.
d. is never associated with problem wounds.

27. Orthostatic blood pressure is defined as:
a. Blood pressure falls 30 mm Hg and the pulse rate increases 10 beats per minute
b. Blood pressure falls 20 mm Hg and the pulse rate increases 10 beats per minute
c. Blood pressure falls 30 mm Hg and the pulse rate increases 30 beats per minute
d. Blood pressure falls 20 mm Hg and the pulse rate increases 20 beats per minute

28. Diabetic patients have an increased risk of which of the following conditions?
a. Osteomyelitis
b. Anemia
c. Compartment syndrome
d. Carbon monoxide poisoning

29. You are performing a neurological examination on a patient with decompression sickness. Which of the following is not part of the examination?

a. Instruct the patient to clench his teeth.
b. Instruct the patient to rub his shin with the heel of the opposite foot.
c. Instruct the patient to bend forward and reach toward his toes.
d. Instruct the patient to touch his nose with his fingertip, while holding his eyes closed.

30. Which of the following statements is NOT true?

a. Treatment for carbon monoxide poisoning aims to reduce hypoxia.
b. Hemoglobin's affinity for oxygen exceeds that for carbon monoxide.
c. Carbon monoxide poisoning can cause long-term neurological damage.
d. Carbon monoxide lowers the amount of oxygen delivered to tissues.

31. The following patients have an increased risk of complications during an HBOT session EXCEPT:

a. Patient who had a recent eye surgery
b. Psychotic patient
c. Patient taking cisplatin
d. Patient who has necrotic lesions

32. Which of the following is a relative contraindication for the use of Nellcor pulse oximeter?

a. Patient who is critical
b. Patient with a respiratory dysfunction
c. Patient with carbon monoxide poisoning
d. There are no contraindications for the use Nellcor pulse oximeter

33. Emergency response care for decompression sickness should include all of the following EXCEPT:

a. Provide the patient 100% oxygen
b. Prevent the patient from drinking
c. Have the patient lie down
d. Keep the patient warm

34. Decompression sickness (DCS) is divided into different types, based on the severity and symptoms. A patient with arterial gas embolism would be classified with which type of DCS?

a. Type 1
b. Type 2
c. Type 3
d. Type 4

35. What does $tcPO_2$ stand for?

a. Transcutaneous Oxygen Module
b. Transcutaneous Oximetry
c. Transcutaneous Oxygen Tension
d. Transcutaneous Oxygen Concentration

36. Which of the following statements is true when using a built-in breathing system (BIBS) during a hyperbaric oxygen therapy?
   a. Reduces the risk of fire
   b. Increases ventilation through the chamber's exhaust valve
   c. Lowers the hyperbaric therapy session duration considerably
   d. Eliminates the need for "air breaks" during the therapy session

37. The National Fire Protection Association (NFPA) classifies a duoplace hyperbaric chamber as a __________ chamber.
   a. Class A
   b. Class B
   c. Class C
   d. Class D

38. You work in a facility located in the United States and receive a pressurized gas cylinder that has a black label. What is the content of the cylinder?
   a. Carbon dioxide
   b. Nitrogen
   c. Nitrous oxide
   d. Oxygen/Nitrogen mixture

39. Which of the following is a typical pre-dive checklist procedure when preparing a chamber for HBOT?
   a. Checking electrical accessories for proper functioning
   b. Evaluating patient's clothing for static properties
   c. Checking the chemical absorbent levels in scrubbers
   d. All the above

40. Which of the following organizations governs the handling of decompressed gases with regard to hyperbaric chambers?
   a. The Occupational Safety and Health Administration (OSHA)
   b. The Food and Drug Administration (FDA)
   c. The Joint Commission
   d. The American Society of Mechanical Engineers (ASME)

41. Which of the following statements is NOT true?
   a. Hyperbaric chamber must be ventilated to maintain required pressure during a therapy session.
   b. Exhaled gases fill the multiplace chamber air, and need to be vented out via release valve in order to reduce fire risk.
   c. In case of possible oxygen toxicity during a hyperbaric oxygen therapy, a patient must be taken off 100% oxygen immediately.
   d. Communication between a patient and staff must be maintained during a hyperbaric oxygen therapy session.

42. Target $tcPO_2$ value for problem wounds, after a hyperbaric oxygen therapy session, is around _______.

a. 40 mm Hg
b. 80 mm Hg
c. 100 mm Hg
d. 200 mm Hg

43. Which of the following statements is NOT true?

a. Hyperbaric chamber fires are most commonly caused by faulty electrical systems.
b. Two patients in a multiplace hyperbaric chamber can be treated with different oxygen therapy protocols.
c. Decompressing a hyperbaric oxygen chamber too quickly can injure people inside and outside the chamber.
d. Multiplace hyperbaric chambers have a higher fire risk than monoplace chambers because of the higher 100% oxygen concentration inside the larger multiplace chamber.

44. Which of the following organizations sets the safety standard that regulates acrylic windows used in hyperbaric chambers?

a. The American Society of Mechanical Engineers (ASME)
b. The National Fire Protection Association (NFPA)
c. The Uniform Boiler and Pressure Vessel Laws Society (UBPVS)
d. The Occupational Safety and Health Administration (OSHA)

Read the following paragraph and answer questions 45 and 46:

You are preparing an unconscious 20-year-old male patient who has a deep and acute laceration in his upper left thigh for a hyperbaric oxygen therapy. You learn that the cause of the laceration is unknown, the laceration was cleaned and sutured on arrival to the emergency department, the patient had blood loss but did not receive a blood transfusion, the patient does not have any underlying medical conditions, his electrocardiogram is abnormal, and he shows signs of breathing distress, pale skin, and low blood pressure.

45. Based on what you know about the patient, what is the most likely reason the patient needs HBOT?

a. Problem wound
b. Anemia
c. Pulmonary embolism
d. Pneumothorax

46. What is your first action in treating this patient?

a. Perform neurological examination.
b. Use Nellcor pulse oximeter to evaluate oxygen levels.
c. Take orthostatic vital signs.
d. All the above.

47. Which of the following increases the risk for barotrauma during hyperbaric oxygen therapy?

a. Diabetes
b. Arthritis
c. Respiratory tract infection
d. None of the above

48. Which of the following statements is NOT true when taking $tcPO_2$ readings?

a. Placing the electrode over a bone can give unreliable results.
b. Waiting less than 15 minutes when taking the tcPO2 readings can cause unreliable results.
c. tcPO2 readings should be taken in a temperature 21° to 23°C.
d. The electrode needs to be in contact with dry skin for reliable readings.

49. You are performing transcutaneous oxygen monitoring (TCOM). What does RPI refer to?

a. Relative Perfusion Index
b. Relative Pressure Index
c. Regional Perfusion Index
d. Regional Pressure Index

50. A blocked artery in the lungs refers to what condition?

a. Nitrogen narcosis
b. Carbon monoxide poisoning
c. Barotrauma
d. Pulmonary embolism

Answers and Explanations

1. A: Henry's law describes the solubility of gases into liquid and is the correct answer. Boyle's law describes the relationship between gas quantity, pressure, volume, and temperature, Charles' law describes the expansion of gases when heated, and Dalton's law describes the partial pressures of gases in a mixture.

2. C: The correct answer is 0.6 atm and can be solved using Dalton's law: $P_x=P_{total}\ (n_x/n_{total})$, where P_x is partial pressure of gas x, P_{total} is total pressure of all gases (1 atm), n_x is the number of moles of gas x, and n_{total} is number of moles of all gases. P_x = 1 atm (0.3 mol/0.5 mol) = 0.6 atm.

3. D: The correct answer is 2.7 L and can be solved using Boyle's law: Vf = PiVi/Pf, where Pi is initial pressure, Vi is initial volume, Pf is final pressure, and Vf is final volume. Pressure of 101.32 kPa = 1 atm. Vf = 3 atm * 0.9 L / 1 atm = 2.7 L.

4. C: Absolute pressure is the combination of water and air pressure acting on a point, and is expressed as atmosphere absolute (atm abs), or ATA. Atmospheric pressure is typically referred to as atm. Gauge pressure is defined as square inch gauge (psig). Partial pressure of oxygen is referred to as PO_2.

5. A: Dalton's law describes partial pressures of gases in a mixture, and is the correct answer. Henry's law describes the solubility of gases into a liquid. Boyle's law describes the relationship between gas quantity, pressure, volume, and temperature. Charles' law describes the expansion of gases when heated.

6. B: The respiratory system is responsible for exchanging carbon dioxide; oxygen needed for cellular respiration is obtained from inhaled air. Respiratory gases are carried in blood and exchanged in the lungs. Respiratory system delivers oxygen to the body tissues and removes carbon dioxide, not carbon monoxide.

7. C: Arteries become progressively smaller as they leave the heart, branching into tissues and delivering oxygen-rich blood to cells. Veins carry blood toward the heart, while arteries carry oxygen-rich blood away from the heart. Veins and arteries connect to heart, while capillaries connect to body tissues. The walls of veins are less thick than the muscular walls of arteries.

8. A: When your body's carbon dioxide level increases, the respiration center in your brain responds by increasing the respiration rate and depth, in order to eliminate excess carbon dioxide from the body. Decreasing the respiration rate and/or depth would reduce the removal of CO_2 from the body.

9. A: People who suffer from hyperthermia (they are overheated) have an increased risk of experiencing oxygen toxicity. Similarly, patients with vitamin E deficiency (not vitamin A) and hyperthyroidism have an increased risk of experiencing oxygen toxicity. Patients with hypothyroidism are actually less likely to suffer from oxygen toxicity.

10. D: Failure to equalize middle ear pressure can lead to middle ear barotrauma. Ascending while exhaling is the proper way to surface. Ascending without exhaling can cause pulmonary barotrauma due to expanding gases. Inhaling while descending does not cause barotrauma since inhaled gases compress, not expand, with increasing depth.

11. B: The "staggers" refers to a nervous system complication of decompression sickness, which affects the inner ear and cerebellum and causes ringing in the ears. Gas bubbles in the pulmonary artery are most likely associated with pulmonary decompression sickness, also known as the "chokes." Purple skin rash is associated with a decompression sickness that affects the skin, also known as the "skin bends."

12. B: Decreased body temperature interferes with metabolism and enzyme function, causing the nervous system and other organs not to work properly. Hypothermia occurs when the body loses heat faster, not slower, than it can produce heat, and causes body temperature to drop below 95°F. Heat stroke is associated with hyperthermia, not hypothermia.

13. C: Embolism can trigger platelets to release clotting factors that eventually lead to blood clotting. This is an acute effect, meaning it can occur very rapidly and within a short time period after the embolism. Whereas, hearing loss, necrosis, and osteonecrosis are chronic or long-term effects of lack of oxygen. These only develop after the tissue has been deprived of oxygen for some time.

14. A: As pressure increases with depth, deep sea diving exerts increased pressure, not decreased, on the body. With increasing depth, more nitrogen dissolves into tissues than at sea level, due to the high pressure exerted on body, whereas breathing pressurized oxygen does not cause nitrogen narcosis. Quick change in the surrounding pressure from high to low causes nitrogen bubbles to enter the bloodstream, leading to decompression sickness, not nitrogen narcosis.

15. C: Diving in cold water, not in warm water, is generally believed to increase the risk of decompression sickness. Dehydration, high body fat, and drinking alcohol before or after a dive can also increase the risk of decompression sickness.

16. A: Scientific studies have not provided evidence to support a claim that hyperbaric oxygen therapy (HBOT) helps patients with arthritis. However, HBOT is approved and recommended for the treatment of arterial gas embolism, delayed radiation injury of the soft tissue or bones, and anemia.

17. A: Transcutaneous oxygen monitoring (TCOM) is used to measure oxygen content of wound tissue to evaluate the level of hypoxia. TCOM measures transcutaneous oxygen tension ($tcPO_2$), and is not used to determine the need for $tcPO_2$. TCOM does not prevent tissue death, but rather evaluates the risk for tissue death.

18. D: Potential complications from hyperbaric oxygen therapy can include seizures caused by too much oxygen in the central nervous system (CNS); organ damage due to air pressure changes (barotrauma); and myopia (temporary nearsightedness) due to increased blood oxygen levels.

19. C: The increased surrounding pressure, generated by hyperbaric oxygen therapy, reduces the size of gas bubbles, such as nitrogen, and decreases the risk of arterial gas embolism. The controlled pressure changes during HBOT causes gases to be released slower, not faster, from the tissue than the rate they are degassed from the body. This helps to eliminate gas bubble formation. There is no mechanism within the body that would limit nitrogen to be carried only in the veins.

20. C: Facial twitching is a sign of CNS oxygen toxicity. Your immediate action should be to take the patient off oxygen to reduce further oxygen toxicity. This should be followed by decompressing the chamber gradually in order to prevent any injuries resulting from rapid decompression. Performing a neurological examination and taking vital signs should be done after decompression.

21. D: The recommended HBOT protocol for nonhealing, problem wounds is one or two 1.5-hour sessions of 100% oxygen at 2 to 2.4 ATA per day.

22. B: Osteoclasts are bone-destroying cells that disrupt and weaken bone tissue. Increasing the number of osteoclasts is not a beneficial effect for treating osteoradionecrosis. However, promoting blood cell and connective tissue formation and increasing tissue oxygen levels (decreasing hypoxia) are beneficial effects of HBOT. These actions promote bone tissue healing, and restore the balance between bone-building cells (osteoblasts) and bone-destroying osteoclasts.

23. C: When treatment for decompression sickness is delayed more than 6 hours, the US Navy Treatment Table 6A recommends recompression to 165 feet for 30 minutes with 50-50 mixture of nitrox or heliox breathing gases.

24. B: SCUBA diving can cause pressure-induced tissue damage also known as barotrauma. This occurs when the diver ascends too fast, surfaces without exhaling, or fails to equalize pressure inside diving mask and ears. Barotrauma can cause 1) pneumothorax associated with breathing difficulties and upper back pain, 2) ear squeeze associated with hearing difficulties, and 3) ocular barotrauma associated with bruising of the eyelids.

25. D: Transcutaneous oxygen monitoring uses a device called transcutaneous oximetry to measure blood oxygen content, or transcutaneous oxygen tension, from outside the body. It is noninvasive method to monitor blood oxygen in newborns and other patients.

26. A: Low tissue oxygen concentration, or hypoxia, increases the likelihood of tissue death. Oxygen toxicity is a result of breathing high concentration of oxygen and does not cause low tissue oxygen. Hypoxic tissues are treated with high-pressure therapy, not high-altitude therapy, which is associated with low oxygen. Problem wounds are always associated with hypoxia.

27. D: A patient is considered to be orthostatic if blood pressure falls 20 mm Hg and pulse rate increases 20 beats per minute.

28. A: Osteomyelitis is a bone infection that can occur when a chronic wound gets infected with a microorganism. Diabetic patients often develop nonhealing wounds, which increase their risk of contracting osteomyelitis. There is no scientific evidence to indicate that

diabetes would increase the risk of anemia, compartment syndrome, or carbon monoxide poisoning.

29. C: Instructing the patient to bend forward and reach for his feet is not part of the neurological examination. Teeth clenching is a part of the face check, and touching the nose and rubbing the shin are part of the coordination check.

30. B: Hemoglobin has a higher affinity toward carbon monoxide than oxygen. This means that when CO is present in blood, hemoglobin binds carbon monoxide over oxygen. Treatment for CO poisoning aims to increase tissue oxygen (decrease hypoxia). CO poisoning can cause neurological damage, and CO lowers the amount of oxygen carried to tissues.

31. D: Hyperbaric oxygen therapy is a recommended treatment form for necrotic wounds and lesions. Patients with recent eye surgery or severe mental disorders such as psychosis, and patients taking cisplatin should not undergo HBOT.

32. C: The use of Nellcor pulse oximeter is contraindicated if a patient suffers from carbon monoxide poisoning because of inaccurate readings. Nellcor pulse oximeter is indicated for critical patients or patients with respiratory dysfunction.

33. B: Emergency response for decompression sickness (DCS) should include providing the patient with 100% oxygen, giving oral or IV fluids to keep the patient hydrated, keeping the patient warm, and having the patient lie down to minimize bubble migration. Preventing the patient from drinking can lead to dehydration and is not a correct emergency response for DCS.

34. C: DCS is divided into type 1, 2 and 3. There is no type 4 DCS. The most severe type of DCS is type 3 and includes patients with arterial gas embolism.

35. C: Transcutaneous oxygen tension is $tcPO_2$. Transcutaneous oxygen module teaches the basics of transcutaneous oxygen monitoring (TCOM). TCOM refers to the techniques needed to measures transcutaneous oxygen tension, or $tcPO_2$, in body tissues.

36. A: Oxygen is highly flammable, and using oxygen increases the risk of fire. Using built-in breathing system (BIBS) allows pure oxygen to be delivered to the patient through a face mask, while the large chamber is filled with air (20% oxygen). This reduces the amount of oxygen used during therapy, which reduces fire risk. Ventilation is maintained via the "overboard dump" system associated with BIBS, the therapy session duration remains unchanged, and air breaks are still needed.

37. A: NFPA classifies duoplace hyperbaric chamber as class A chamber.

38. B: In the United States, color coding indicating nitrogen is black, carbon dioxide is gray, nitrous oxide is blue, and oxygen/nitrogen mixtures are either yellow or black and green, depending on the oxygen concentration.

39. D: All these procedures are included in the pre-dive checklist. Before performing a HBOT, the hyperbaric technologist should check all electrical accessories for possible problems that could cause a fire hazard. The technologist should also check scrubbers for

absorbent, and ensure that the patient is wearing clothing made of nonstatic materials to decrease fire risk.

40. A: The use and handling of compressed gases used in hyperbaric chambers is governed by the Occupational Safety and Health Administration under the rule 1910.101 parts a, b, and c.

41. B: Exhaled gases are removed via individual masks, which also supply the breathing gases, in multiplace chambers. In monoplace chambers, which can be operated without individual BIBS masks, the oxygen-rich atmosphere needs to be removed via release valve.

42. D: The target tissue $tcPO_2$ value is 200 mm Hg for hyperbaric oxygen therapy patients who have problem wounds.

43. D: Multiplace chambers use individual face masks, or BIBS, to deliver oxygen to patients. This reduces the use of oxygen as the remaining chamber is filled with air. High fire risk associated with HBOT is due to high oxygen use.

44. A: Acrylic windows used in hyperbaric chambers are regulated by PVHO-1 safety standard set by the ASME. The NFPA Standard 99, Chapter 19 requires that hyperbaric chambers are designed following the ASME PVOH-1 standard, and the UBPVS is part of ASME and promotes national ASME standards for boilers and pressure vessels.

45. B: Based on the patient history, the most logical diagnosis is anemia due to severe blood loss, caused by a traumatic injury. When a patient who has lost large quantity of blood does not receive a blood transfusion, it can cause a condition known as blood loss anemia. HBOT is used to oxygenate tissues until blood transfusion becomes available, or the patient does not suffer from hypoxia anymore. Problem wound is a chronic, necrotic wound, and is not sutured. Pulmonary embolism is generally caused by a blood clot that blocks blood flow in the lungs. Although some of the symptoms are similar (breathing distress and low blood pressure), unless there is reason to suspect the condition is caused by gas bubbles (after a dive), hyperbaric oxygen therapy is not used to treat the condition. Based on the patient history, there is no reason to think the patient suffers from pulmonary embolism or pneumothorax (collapsed lung).

46. B: Nellcor pulse oximeter measures blood oxygen content and is typically used to monitor oxygen levels on a critical patient. Neurological examination is contraindicated in unconscious patients. Orthostatic vital signs should be taken from a nontrauma patient with suspected hypovolemia, but cannot be taken from an unconscious patient.

47. C: Respiratory tract infection, such as cold, causes congestion, which can lead to inability to equalize pressure in the ear. This increased pressure can lead to a middle ear barotrauma during a HBOT session. Diabetes or arthritis does not increase the risk of barotrauma during a HBOT session.

48. D: There needs to be liquid between the electrode and skin to get reliable $tcPO_2$ readings. Contact liquid, or gel, needs to be used in order to prevent an air pocket between the skin and the electrode. Placing the electrode over a bone, taking readings in cooler or warmer ambient temperature than room temperature, and waiting less than 15 minutes to take the reading can cause unreliable results.

49. C: TCOM refers to transcutaneous oxygen monitoring, which evaluates tissue oxygen content or tension ($tcPO_2$) using a transcutaneous oximetry. RPI refers to regional perfusion index. RPI can be calculated using a computer program and the $tcPO_2$ results obtained from the patient.

50. D: A blocked artery in the lungs refers to pulmonary embolism, which is caused by a gas bubble or a blood clot that blocks a blood vessel in the lungs. Nitrogen narcosis refers to increased levels of nitrogen in the body, which causes confusion and impairment. Carbon monoxide poisoning refers to increased levels of carbon monoxide in the body. Barotrauma refers to a tissue injury caused by high pressure.

Secret Key #1 - Time is Your Greatest Enemy

Pace Yourself

Wear a watch. At the beginning of the test, check the time (or start a chronometer on your watch to count the minutes), and check the time after every few questions to make sure you are "on schedule."

If you are forced to speed up, do it efficiently. Usually one or more answer choices can be eliminated without too much difficulty. Above all, don't panic. Don't speed up and just begin guessing at random choices. By pacing yourself, and continually monitoring your progress against your watch, you will always know exactly how far ahead or behind you are with your available time. If you find that you are one minute behind on the test, don't skip one question without spending any time on it, just to catch back up. Take 15 fewer seconds on the next four questions, and after four questions you'll have caught back up. Once you catch back up, you can continue working each problem at your normal pace.

Furthermore, don't dwell on the problems that you were rushed on. If a problem was taking up too much time and you made a hurried guess, it must be difficult. The difficult questions are the ones you are most likely to miss anyway, so it isn't a big loss. It is better to end with more time than you need than to run out of time.

Lastly, sometimes it is beneficial to slow down if you are constantly getting ahead of time. You are always more likely to catch a careless mistake by working more slowly than quickly, and among very high-scoring test takers (those who are likely to have lots of time left over), careless errors affect the score more than mastery of material.

Secret Key #2 - Guessing is not Guesswork

You probably know that guessing is a good idea. Unlike other standardized tests, there is no penalty for getting a wrong answer. Even if you have no idea about a question, you still have a 20-25% chance of getting it right.

Most test takers do not understand the impact that proper guessing can have on their score. Unless you score extremely high, guessing will significantly contribute to your final score.

Monkeys Take the Test

What most test takers don't realize is that to insure that 20-25% chance, you have to guess randomly. If you put 20 monkeys in a room to take this test, assuming they answered once per question and behaved themselves, on average they would get 20-25% of the questions correct. Put 20 test takers in the room, and the average will be much lower among guessed questions. Why?

1. The test writers intentionally write deceptive answer choices that "look" right. A test

taker has no idea about a question, so he picks the "best looking" answer, which is often wrong. The monkey has no idea what looks good and what doesn't, so it will consistently be right about 20-25% of the time.

2. Test takers will eliminate answer choices from the guessing pool based on a hunch or intuition. Simple but correct answers often get excluded, leaving a 0% chance of being correct. The monkey has no clue, and often gets lucky with the best choice.

This is why the process of elimination endorsed by most test courses is flawed and detrimental to your performance. Test takers don't guess; they make an ignorant stab in the dark that is usually worse than random.

$5 Challenge

Let me introduce one of the most valuable ideas of this course—the $5 challenge:

You only mark your "best guess" if you are willing to bet $5 on it.
You only eliminate choices from guessing if you are willing to bet $5 on it.

Why $5? Five dollars is an amount of money that is small yet not insignificant, and can really add up fast (20 questions could cost you $100). Likewise, each answer choice on one question of the test will have a small impact on your overall score, but it can really add up to a lot of points in the end.

The process of elimination IS valuable. The following shows your chance of guessing it right:

If you eliminate wrong answer choices until only this many remain:	Chance of getting it correct:
1	100%
2	50%
3	33%

However, if you accidentally eliminate the right answer or go on a hunch for an incorrect answer, your chances drop dramatically—to 0%. By guessing among all the answer choices, you are GUARANTEED to have a shot at the right answer.

That's why the $5 test is so valuable. If you give up the advantage and safety of a pure guess, it had better be worth the risk.

What we still haven't covered is how to be sure that whatever guess you make is truly random. Here's the easiest way:

Always pick the first answer choice among those remaining.

Such a technique means that you have decided, **before you see a single test question**, exactly how you are going to guess, and since the order of choices tells you nothing about which one is correct, this guessing technique is perfectly random.

This section is not meant to scare you away from making educated guesses or eliminating choices; you just need to define when a choice is worth eliminating. The $5 test, along with a pre-defined random guessing strategy, is the best way to make sure you reap all of the benefits of guessing.

Secret Key #3 - Practice Smarter, Not Harder

Many test takers delay the test preparation process because they dread the awful amounts of practice time they think necessary to succeed on the test. We have refined an effective method that will take you only a fraction of the time.

There are a number of "obstacles" in the path to success. Among these are answering questions, finishing in time, and mastering test-taking strategies. All must be executed on the day of the test at peak performance, or your score will suffer. The test is a mental marathon that has a large impact on your future.

Just like a marathon runner, it is important to work your way up to the full challenge. So first you just worry about questions, and then time, and finally strategy:

Success Strategy

1. Find a good source for practice tests.
2. If you are willing to make a larger time investment, consider using more than one study guide. Often the different approaches of multiple authors will help you "get" difficult concepts.
3. Take a practice test with no time constraints, with all study helps, "open book." Take your time with questions and focus on applying strategies.
4. Take a practice test with time constraints, with all guides, "open book."
5. Take a final practice test without open material and with time limits.

If you have time to take more practice tests, just repeat step 5. By gradually exposing yourself to the full rigors of the test environment, you will condition your mind to the stress of test day and maximize your success.

Secret Key #4 - Prepare, Don't Procrastinate

Let me state an obvious fact: if you take the test three times, you will probably get three different scores. This is due to the way you feel on test day, the level of preparedness you have, and the version of the test you see. Despite the test writers' claims to the contrary, some versions of the test WILL be easier for you than others.

Since your future depends so much on your score, you should maximize your chances of success. In order to maximize the likelihood of success, you've got to prepare in advance.

This means taking practice tests and spending time learning the information and test taking strategies you will need to succeed.

Never go take the actual test as a "practice" test, expecting that you can just take it again if you need to. Take all the practice tests you can on your own, but when you go to take the official test, be prepared, be focused, and do your best the first time!

Secret Key #5 - Test Yourself

Everyone knows that time is money. There is no need to spend too much of your time or too little of your time preparing for the test. You should only spend as much of your precious time preparing as is necessary for you to get the score you need.

Once you have taken a practice test under real conditions of time constraints, then you will know if you are ready for the test or not.

If you have scored extremely high the first time that you take the practice test, then there is not much point in spending countless hours studying. You are already there.

Benchmark your abilities by retaking practice tests and seeing how much you have improved. Once you consistently score high enough to guarantee success, then you are ready.

If you have scored well below where you need, then knuckle down and begin studying in earnest. Check your improvement regularly through the use of practice tests under real conditions. Above all, don't worry, panic, or give up. The key is perseverance!

Then, when you go to take the test, remain confident and remember how well you did on the practice tests. If you can score high enough on a practice test, then you can do the same on the real thing.

General Strategies

The most important thing you can do is to ignore your fears and jump into the test immediately. Do not be overwhelmed by any strange-sounding terms. You have to jump into the test like jumping into a pool—all at once is the easiest way.

Make Predictions

As you read and understand the question, try to guess what the answer will be. Remember that several of the answer choices are wrong, and once you begin reading them, your mind will immediately become cluttered with answer choices designed to throw you off. Your mind is typically the most focused immediately after you have read the question and digested its contents. If you can, try to predict what the correct answer will be. You may be surprised at what you can predict.

Quickly scan the choices and see if your prediction is in the listed answer choices. If it is, then you can be quite confident that you have the right answer. It still won't hurt to check the other answer choices, but most of the time, you've got it!

Answer the Question

It may seem obvious to only pick answer choices that answer the question, but the test writers can create some excellent answer choices that are wrong. Don't pick an answer just because it sounds right, or you believe it to be true. It MUST answer the question. Once you've made your selection, always go back and check it against the question and make sure that you didn't misread the question and that the answer choice does answer the question posed.

Benchmark

After you read the first answer choice, decide if you think it sounds correct or not. If it doesn't, move on to the next answer choice. If it does, mentally mark that answer choice. This doesn't mean that you've definitely selected it as your answer choice, it just means that it's the best you've seen thus far. Go ahead and read the next choice. If the next choice is worse than the one you've already selected, keep going to the next answer choice. If the next choice is better than the choice you've already selected, mentally mark the new answer choice as your best guess.

The first answer choice that you select becomes your standard. Every other answer choice must be benchmarked against that standard. That choice is correct until proven otherwise by another answer choice beating it out. Once you've decided that no other answer choice seems as good, do one final check to ensure that your answer choice answers the question posed.

Valid Information

Don't discount any of the information provided in the question. Every piece of information may be necessary to determine the correct answer. None of the information in the question is there to throw you off (while the answer choices will certainly have information to throw you off). If two seemingly unrelated topics are discussed, don't ignore either. You can be confident there is a relationship, or it wouldn't be included in the question, and you are probably going to have to determine what is that relationship to find the answer.

Avoid "Fact Traps"

Don't get distracted by a choice that is factually true. Your search is for the answer that answers the question. Stay focused and don't fall for an answer that is true but irrelevant. Always go back to the question and make sure you're choosing an answer that actually answers the question and is not just a true statement. An answer can be factually correct, but it MUST answer the question asked. Additionally, two answers can both be seemingly correct, so be sure to read all of the answer choices, and make sure that you get the one that BEST answers the question.

Milk the Question

Some of the questions may throw you completely off. They might deal with a subject you have not been exposed to, or one that you haven't reviewed in years. While your lack of knowledge about the subject will be a hindrance, the question itself can give you many clues that will help you find the correct answer. Read the question carefully and look for clues. Watch particularly for adjectives and nouns describing difficult terms or words that you don't recognize. Regardless of whether you completely understand a word or not, replacing it with a synonym, either provided or one you more familiar with, may help you to understand what the questions are asking. Rather than wracking your mind about specific detailed information concerning a difficult term or word, try to use mental substitutes that are easier to understand.

The Trap of Familiarity

Don't just choose a word because you recognize it. On difficult questions, you may not recognize a number of words in the answer choices. The test writers don't put "make-believe" words on the test, so don't think that just because you only recognize all the words in one answer choice that that answer choice must be correct. If you only recognize words in one answer choice, then focus on that one. Is it correct? Try your best to determine if it is correct. If it is, that's great. If not, eliminate it. Each word and answer choice you eliminate increases your chances of getting the question correct, even if you then have to guess among the unfamiliar choices.

Eliminate Answers

Eliminate choices as soon as you realize they are wrong. But be careful! Make sure you consider all of the possible answer choices. Just because one appears right, doesn't mean that the next one won't be even better! The test writers will usually put more than one good answer choice for every question, so read all of them. Don't worry if you are stuck between two that seem right. By getting down to just two remaining possible choices, your odds are now 50/50. Rather than wasting too much time, play the odds. You are guessing, but guessing wisely because you've been able to knock out some of the answer choices that you know are wrong. If you are eliminating choices and realize that the last answer choice you are left with is also obviously wrong, don't panic. Start over and consider each choice again. There may easily be something that you missed the first time and will realize on the second pass.

Tough Questions

If you are stumped on a problem or it appears too hard or too difficult, don't waste time. Move on! Remember though, if you can quickly check for obviously incorrect answer choices, your chances of guessing correctly are greatly improved. Before you completely give up, at least try to knock out a couple of possible answers. Eliminate what you can and then guess at the remaining answer choices before moving on.

Brainstorm

If you get stuck on a difficult question, spend a few seconds quickly brainstorming. Run through the complete list of possible answer choices. Look at each choice and ask yourself, "Could this answer the question satisfactorily?" Go through each answer choice and consider it independently of the others. By systematically going through all possibilities, you may find something that you would otherwise overlook. Remember though that when you get stuck, it's important to try to keep moving.

Read Carefully

Understand the problem. Read the question and answer choices carefully. Don't miss the question because you misread the terms. You have plenty of time to read each question thoroughly and make sure you understand what is being asked. Yet a happy medium must be attained, so don't waste too much time. You must read carefully, but efficiently.

Face Value

When in doubt, use common sense. Always accept the situation in the problem at face value. Don't read too much into it. These problems will not require you to make huge leaps of logic. The test writers aren't trying to throw you off with a cheap trick. If you have to go beyond creativity and make a leap of logic in order to have an answer choice answer the question, then you should look at the other answer choices. Don't overcomplicate the problem by creating theoretical relationships or explanations that will warp time or space. These are normal problems rooted in reality. It's just that the applicable relationship or explanation may not be readily apparent and you have to figure things out. Use your common sense to interpret anything that isn't clear.

Prefixes

If you're having trouble with a word in the question or answer choices, try dissecting it. Take advantage of every clue that the word might include. Prefixes and suffixes can be a huge help. Usually they allow you to determine a basic meaning. Pre- means before, post- means after, pro - is positive, de- is negative. From these prefixes and suffixes, you can get an idea of the general meaning of the word and try to put it into context. Beware though of any traps. Just because con- is the opposite of pro-, doesn't necessarily mean congress is the opposite of progress!

Hedge Phrases

Watch out for critical hedge phrases, led off with words such as "likely," "may," "can," "sometimes," "often," "almost," "mostly," "usually," "generally," "rarely," and "sometimes." Question writers insert these hedge phrases to cover every possibility. Often an answer choice will be wrong simply because it leaves no room for exception. Unless the situation calls for them, avoid answer choices that have definitive words like "exactly," and "always."

Switchback Words

Stay alert for "switchbacks." These are the words and phrases frequently used to alert you to shifts in thought. The most common switchback word is "but." Others include "although," "however," "nevertheless," "on the other hand," "even though," "while," "in spite of," "despite," and "regardless of."

New Information

Correct answer choices will rarely have completely new information included. Answer choices typically are straightforward reflections of the material asked about and will directly relate to the question. If a new piece of information is included in an answer choice that doesn't even seem to relate to the topic being asked about, then that answer choice is likely incorrect. All of the information needed to answer the question is usually provided for you in the question. You should not have to make guesses that are unsupported or choose answer choices that require unknown information that cannot be reasoned from what is given.

Time Management

On technical questions, don't get lost on the technical terms. Don't spend too much time on any one question. If you don't know what a term means, then odds are you aren't going to get much further since you don't have a dictionary. You should be able to immediately recognize whether or not you know a term. If you don't, work with the other clues that you have—the other answer choices and terms provided—but don't waste too much time trying to figure out a difficult term that you don't know.

Contextual Clues

Look for contextual clues. An answer can be right but not the correct answer. The contextual clues will help you find the answer that is most right and is correct. Understand the context in which a phrase or statement is made. This will help you make important distinctions.

Don't Panic

Panicking will not answer any questions for you; therefore, it isn't helpful. When you first see the question, if your mind goes blank, take a deep breath. Force yourself to mechanically go through the steps of solving the problem using the strategies you've learned.

Pace Yourself

Don't get clock fever. It's easy to be overwhelmed when you're looking at a page full of questions, your mind is full of random thoughts and feeling confused, and the clock is ticking down faster than you would like. Calm down and maintain the pace that you have set for yourself. As long as you are on track by monitoring your pace, you are guaranteed to have enough time for yourself. When you get to the last few minutes of the test, it may seem like you won't have enough time left, but if you only have as many questions as you should have left at that point, then you're right on track!

Answer Selection

The best way to pick an answer choice is to eliminate all of those that are wrong, until only one is left and confirm that is the correct answer. Sometimes though, an answer choice may immediately look right. Be careful! Take a second to make sure that the other choices are not equally obvious. Don't make a hasty mistake. There are only two times that you should stop before checking other answers. First is when you are positive that the answer choice you have selected is correct. Second is when time is almost out and you have to make a quick guess!

Check Your Work

Since you will probably not know every term listed and the answer to every question, it is important that you get credit for the ones that you do know. Don't miss any questions through careless mistakes. If at all possible, try to take a second to look back over your answer selection and make sure you've selected the correct answer choice and haven't made a costly careless mistake (such as marking an answer choice that you didn't mean to mark). The time it takes for this quick double check should more than pay for itself in caught mistakes.

Beware of Directly Quoted Answers

Sometimes an answer choice will repeat word for word a portion of the question or reference section. However, beware of such exact duplication. It may be a trap! More than likely, the correct choice will paraphrase or summarize a point, rather than being exactly the same wording.

Slang

Scientific sounding answers are better than slang ones. An answer choice that begins "To compare the outcomes..." is much more likely to be correct than one that begins "Because some people insisted..."

Extreme Statements

Avoid wild answers that throw out highly controversial ideas that are proclaimed as established fact. An answer choice that states the "process should used in certain situations, if..." is much more likely to be correct than one that states the "process should be discontinued completely." The first is a calm rational statement and doesn't even make a definitive, uncompromising stance, using a hedge word "if" to provide wiggle room, whereas the second choice is a radical idea and far more extreme.

Answer Choice Families

When you have two or more answer choices that are direct opposites or parallels, one of them is usually the correct answer. For instance, if one answer choice states "x increases" and another answer choice states "x decreases" or "y increases," then those two or three answer choices are very similar in construction and fall into the same family of answer choices. A family of answer choices consists of two or three answer choices, very similar in construction, but often with directly opposite meanings. Usually the correct answer choice will be in that family of answer choices. The "odd man out" or answer choice that doesn't seem to fit the parallel construction of the other answer choices is more likely to be incorrect.

Special Report: How to Overcome Test Anxiety

The very nature of tests caters to some level of anxiety, nervousness, or tension, just as we feel for any important event that occurs in our lives. A little bit of anxiety or nervousness can be a good thing. It helps us with motivation, and makes achievement just that much sweeter. However, too much anxiety can be a problem, especially if it hinders our ability to function and perform.

"Test anxiety," is the term that refers to the emotional reactions that some test-takers experience when faced with a test or exam. Having a fear of testing and exams is based upon a rational fear, since the test-taker's performance can shape the course of an academic career. Nevertheless, experiencing excessive fear of examinations will only interfere with the test-taker's ability to perform and chance to be successful.

There are a large variety of causes that can contribute to the development and sensation of test anxiety. These include, but are not limited to, lack of preparation and worrying about issues surrounding the test.

Lack of Preparation

Lack of preparation can be identified by the following behaviors or situations:

Not scheduling enough time to study, and therefore cramming the night before the test or exam
Managing time poorly, to create the sensation that there is not enough time to do everything
Failing to organize the text information in advance, so that the study material consists of the entire text and not simply the pertinent information
Poor overall studying habits

Worrying, on the other hand, can be related to both the test taker, or many other factors around him/her that will be affected by the results of the test. These include worrying about:

Previous performances on similar exams, or exams in general
How friends and other students are achieving
The negative consequences that will result from a poor grade or failure

There are three primary elements to test anxiety. Physical components, which involve the same typical bodily reactions as those to acute anxiety (to be discussed below). Emotional factors have to do with fear or panic. Mental or cognitive issues concerning attention spans and memory abilities.

Physical Signals

There are many different symptoms of test anxiety, and these are not limited to mental and emotional strain. Frequently there are a range of physical signals that will let a test taker know that he/she is suffering from test anxiety. These bodily changes can include the following:

Perspiring
Sweaty palms
Wet, trembling hands
Nausea
Dry mouth
A knot in the stomach
Headache
Faintness
Muscle tension
Aching shoulders, back and neck
Rapid heart beat
Feeling too hot/cold

To recognize the sensation of test anxiety, a test-taker should monitor him/herself for the following sensations:

The physical distress symptoms as listed above
Emotional sensitivity, expressing emotional feelings such as the need to cry or laugh too much, or a sensation of anger or helplessness
A decreased ability to think, causing the test-taker to blank out or have racing thoughts that are hard to organize or control.

Though most students will feel some level of anxiety when faced with a test or exam, the majority can cope with that anxiety and maintain it at a manageable level. However, those who cannot are faced with a very real and very serious condition, which can and should be controlled for the immeasurable benefit of this sufferer.

Naturally, these sensations lead to negative results for the testing experience. The most common effects of test anxiety have to do with nervousness and mental blocking.

Nervousness

Nervousness can appear in several different levels:

The test-taker's difficulty, or even inability to read and understand the questions on the test
The difficulty or inability to organize thoughts to a coherent form
The difficulty or inability to recall key words and concepts relating to the testing questions (especially essays)
The receipt of poor grades on a test, though the test material was well known by the test taker

Conversely, a person may also experience mental blocking, which involves:

Blanking out on test questions
Only remembering the correct answers to the questions when the test has already finished.

Fortunately for test anxiety sufferers, beating these feelings, to a large degree, has to do with proper preparation. When a test taker has a feeling of preparedness, then anxiety will be dramatically lessened.

The first step to resolving anxiety issues is to distinguish which of the two types of anxiety are being suffered. If the anxiety is a direct result of a lack of preparation, this should be considered a normal reaction, and the anxiety level (as opposed to the test results) shouldn't be anything to worry about. However, if, when adequately prepared, the test-taker still panics, blanks out, or seems to overreact, this is not a fully rational reaction. While this can be considered normal too, there are many ways to combat and overcome these effects.

Remember that anxiety cannot be entirely eliminated, however, there are ways to minimize it, to make the anxiety easier to manage. Preparation is one of the best ways to minimize test anxiety. Therefore the following techniques are wise in order to best fight off any anxiety that may want to build.

To begin with, try to avoid cramming before a test, whenever it is possible. By trying to memorize an entire term's worth of information in one day, you'll be shocking your system, and not giving yourself a very good chance to absorb the information. This is an easy path to anxiety, so for those who suffer from test anxiety, cramming should not even be considered an option.

Instead of cramming, work throughout the semester to combine all of the material which is presented throughout the semester, and work on it gradually as the course goes by, making sure to master the main concepts first, leaving minor details for a week or so before the test.

To study for the upcoming exam, be sure to pose questions that may be on the examination, to gauge the ability to answer them by integrating the ideas from your texts, notes and lectures, as well as any supplementary readings.

If it is truly impossible to cover all of the information that was covered in that particular term, concentrate on the most important portions, that can be covered very well. Learn these concepts as best as possible, so that when the test comes, a goal can be made to use these concepts as presentations of your knowledge.

In addition to study habits, changes in attitude are critical to beating a struggle with test anxiety. In fact, an improvement of the perspective over the entire test-taking experience can actually help a test taker to enjoy studying and therefore improve the overall experience. Be certain not to overemphasize the significance of the grade - know that the result of the test is neither a reflection of self worth, nor is it a measure of intelligence; one grade will not predict a person's future success.

To improve an overall testing outlook, the following steps should be tried:

Keeping in mind that the most reasonable expectation for taking a test is to expect to try to demonstrate as much of what you know as you possibly can.
Reminding ourselves that a test is only one test; this is not the only one, and there will be others.
The thought of thinking of oneself in an irrational, all-or-nothing term should be avoided at all costs.
A reward should be designated for after the test, so there's something to look forward to. Whether it be going to a movie, going out to eat, or simply visiting friends, schedule it in advance, and do it no matter what result is expected on the exam.

Test-takers should also keep in mind that the basics are some of the most important things, even beyond anti-anxiety techniques and studying. Never neglect the basic social, emotional and biological needs, in order to try to absorb information. In order to best achieve, these three factors must be held as just as important as the studying itself.

Study Steps

Remember the following important steps for studying:

Maintain healthy nutrition and exercise habits. Continue both your recreational activities and social pass times. These both contribute to your physical and emotional well being.
Be certain to get a good amount of sleep, especially the night before the test, because when you're overtired you are not able to perform to the best of your best ability.
Keep the studying pace to a moderate level by taking breaks when they are needed, and varying the work whenever possible, to keep the mind fresh instead of getting bored.
When enough studying has been done that all the material that can be learned has been learned, and the test taker is prepared for the test, stop studying and do something relaxing such as listening to music, watching a movie, or taking a warm bubble bath.

There are also many other techniques to minimize the uneasiness or apprehension that is experienced along with test anxiety before, during, or even after the examination. In fact, there are a great deal of things that can be done to stop anxiety from interfering with lifestyle and performance. Again, remember that anxiety will not be eliminated entirely, and it shouldn't be. Otherwise that "up" feeling for exams would not exist, and most of us depend on that sensation to perform better than usual. However, this anxiety has to be at a level that is manageable.

Of course, as we have just discussed, being prepared for the exam is half the battle right away. Attending all classes, finding out what knowledge will be expected on the exam, and knowing the exam schedules are easy steps to lowering anxiety. Keeping up with work will remove the need to cram, and efficient study habits will eliminate wasted time. Studying should be done in an ideal location for concentration, so that it is simple to become interested in the material and give it complete attention. A method such as SQ3R (Survey, Question, Read, Recite, Review) is a wonderful key to follow to make sure that the study habits are as effective as possible, especially in the case of learning from a textbook. Flashcards are great techniques for memorization. Learning to take good notes will mean that notes will be full of useful information, so that less sifting will need to be done to seek out what is pertinent for studying. Reviewing notes after class and then again on occasion will keep the information fresh in the mind. From notes that have been taken summary sheets and outlines can be made for simpler reviewing.

A study group can also be a very motivational and helpful place to study, as there will be a sharing of ideas, all of the minds can work together, to make sure that everyone understands, and the studying will be made more interesting because it will be a social occasion.

Basically, though, as long as the test-taker remains organized and self confident, with efficient study habits, less time will need to be spent studying, and higher grades will be achieved.

To become self confident, there are many useful steps. The first of these is "self talk." It has been shown through extensive research, that self-talk for students who suffer from test anxiety, should be well monitored, in order to make sure that it contributes to self confidence as opposed to sinking the student. Frequently the self talk of test-anxious students is negative or self-defeating, thinking that everyone else is smarter and faster, that they always mess up, and that if they don't do well, they'll fail the entire course. It is important to decreasing anxiety that awareness is made of self talk. Try writing any negative self thoughts and then disputing them with a positive statement instead. Begin self-encouragement as though it was a friend speaking. Repeat positive statements to help reprogram the mind to believing in successes instead of failures.

Helpful Techniques

Other extremely helpful techniques include:

Self-visualization of doing well and reaching goals
While aiming for an "A" level of understanding, don't try to "overprotect" by setting your expectations lower. This will only convince the mind to stop studying in order to meet the lower expectations.
Don't make comparisons with the results or habits of other students. These are individual factors, and different things work for different people, causing different results.
Strive to become an expert in learning what works well, and what can be done in order to improve. Consider collecting this data in a journal.
Create rewards for after studying instead of doing things before studying that will only turn into avoidance behaviors.
Make a practice of relaxing - by using methods such as progressive relaxation, self-hypnosis, guided imagery, etc - in order to make relaxation an automatic sensation.
Work on creating a state of relaxed concentration so that concentrating will take on the focus of the mind, so that none will be wasted on worrying.
Take good care of the physical self by eating well and getting enough sleep.
Plan in time for exercise and stick to this plan.

Beyond these techniques, there are other methods to be used before, during and after the test that will help the test-taker perform well in addition to overcoming anxiety.

Before the exam comes the academic preparation. This involves establishing a study schedule and beginning at least one week before the actual date of the test. By doing this, the anxiety of not having enough time to study for the test will be automatically eliminated. Moreover, this will make the studying a much more effective experience, ensuring that the learning will be an easier process. This relieves much undue pressure on the test-taker.

Summary sheets, note cards, and flash cards with the main concepts and examples of these main concepts should be prepared in advance of the actual studying time. A topic should never be eliminated from this process. By omitting a topic because it isn't expected to be on the test is only setting up the test-taker for anxiety should it actually appear on the exam. Utilize the course syllabus for laying out the topics that should be studied. Carefully go over the notes that were made in class, paying special attention to any of the issues that the professor took special care to emphasize while lecturing in class. In the textbooks, use the chapter review, or if possible, the chapter tests, to begin your review.

It may even be possible to ask the instructor what information will be covered on the exam, or what the format of the exam will be (for example, multiple choice, essay, free form, true-false). Additionally, see if it is possible to find out how many questions will be on the test. If a review sheet or sample test has been offered by the professor, make good use of it, above anything else, for the preparation for the test. Another great resource for getting to know the examination is reviewing tests from previous semesters. Use these tests to review, and aim to achieve a 100% score on each of the possible topics. With a few exceptions, the goal that you set for yourself is the highest one that you will reach.

Take all of the questions that were assigned as homework, and rework them to any other possible course material. The more problems reworked, the more skill and confidence will form as a result. When forming the solution to a problem, write out each of the steps. Don't simply do head work. By doing as many steps on paper as possible, much clarification and therefore confidence will be formed. Do this with as many homework problems as possible, before checking the answers. By checking the answer after each problem, a reinforcement will exist, that will not be on the exam. Study situations should be as exam-like as possible, to prime the test-taker's system for the experience. By waiting to check the answers at the end, a psychological advantage will be formed, to decrease the stress factor.

Another fantastic reason for not cramming is the avoidance of confusion in concepts, especially when it comes to mathematics. 8-10 hours of study will become one hundred percent more effective if it is spread out over a week or at least several days, instead of doing it all in one sitting. Recognize that the human brain requires time in order to assimilate new material, so frequent breaks and a span of study time over several days will be much more beneficial.

Additionally, don't study right up until the point of the exam. Studying should stop a minimum of one hour before the exam begins. This allows the brain to rest and put things in their proper order. This will also provide the time to become as relaxed as possible when going into the examination room. The test-taker will also have time to eat well and eat sensibly. Know that the brain needs food as much as the rest of the body. With enough food and enough sleep, as well as a relaxed attitude, the body and the mind are primed for success.

Avoid any anxious classmates who are talking about the exam. These students only spread anxiety, and are not worth sharing the anxious sentimentalities.

Before the test also involves creating a positive attitude, so mental preparation should also be a point of concentration. There are many keys to creating a positive attitude. Should fears become rushing in, make a visualization of taking the exam, doing well, and seeing an A written on the paper. Write out a list of affirmations that will bring a feeling of confidence, such as "I am doing well in my English class," "I studied well and know my material," "I enjoy this class." Even if the affirmations aren't believed at first, it sends a positive message to the subconscious which will result in an alteration of the overall belief system, which is the system that creates reality.

If a sensation of panic begins, work with the fear and imagine the very worst! Work through the entire scenario of not passing the test, failing the entire course, and dropping out of school, followed by not getting a job, and pushing a shopping cart through the dark alley where you'll live. This will place things into perspective! Then, practice deep breathing and create a visualization of the opposite situation - achieving an "A" on the exam, passing the entire course, receiving the degree at a graduation ceremony.

On the day of the test, there are many things to be done to ensure the best results, as well as the most calm outlook. The following stages are suggested in order to maximize test-taking potential:

Begin the examination day with a moderate breakfast, and avoid any coffee or beverages with caffeine if the test taker is prone to jitters. Even people who are used to managing caffeine can feel jittery or light-headed when it is taken on a test day.
Attempt to do something that is relaxing before the examination begins. As last minute cramming clouds the mastering of overall concepts, it is better to use this time to create a calming outlook.
Be certain to arrive at the test location well in advance, in order to provide time to select a location that is away from doors, windows and other distractions, as well as giving enough time to relax before the test begins.
Keep away from anxiety generating classmates who will upset the sensation of stability and relaxation that is being attempted before the exam.
Should the waiting period before the exam begins cause anxiety, create a self-distraction by reading.a light magazine or something else that is relaxing and simple.

During the exam itself, read the entire exam from beginning to end, and find out how much time should be allotted to each individual problem. Once writing the exam, should more time be taken for a problem, it should be abandoned, in order to begin another problem. If there is time at the end, the unfinished problem can always be returned to and completed.

Read the instructions very carefully - twice - so that unpleasant surprises won't follow during or after the exam has ended.

When writing the exam, pretend that the situation is actually simply the completion of homework within a library, or at home. This will assist in forming a relaxed atmosphere, and will allow the brain extra focus for the complex thinking function.

Begin the exam with all of the questions with which the most confidence is felt. This will build the confidence level regarding the entire exam and will begin a quality momentum. This will also create encouragement for trying the problems where uncertainty resides.

Going with the "gut instinct" is always the way to go when solving a problem. Second guessing should be avoided at all costs. Have confidence in the ability to do well.

For essay questions, create an outline in advance that will keep the mind organized and make certain that all of the points are remembered. For multiple choice, read every answer, even if the correct one has been spotted - a better one may exist.

Continue at a pace that is reasonable and not rushed, in order to be able to work carefully. Provide enough time to go over the answers at the end, to check for small errors that can be corrected.

Should a feeling of panic begin, breathe deeply, and think of the feeling of the body releasing sand through its pores. Visualize a calm, peaceful place, and include all of the sights, sounds and sensations of this image. Continue the deep breathing, and take a few minutes to continue this with closed eyes. When all is well again, return to the test.

If a "blanking" occurs for a certain question, skip it and move on to the next question. There will be time to return to the other question later. Get everything done that can be done, first, to guarantee all the grades that can be compiled, and to build all of the confidence possible. Then return to the weaker questions to build the marks from there.

Remember, one's own reality can be created, so as long as the belief is there, success will follow. And remember: anxiety can happen later, right now, there's an exam to be written!

After the examination is complete, whether there is a feeling for a good grade or a bad grade, don't dwell on the exam, and be certain to follow through on the reward that was promised...and enjoy it! Don't dwell on any mistakes that have been made, as there is nothing that can be done at this point anyway.

Additionally, don't begin to study for the next test right away. Do something relaxing for a while, and let the mind relax and prepare itself to begin absorbing information again.

From the results of the exam - both the grade and the entire experience, be certain to learn from what has gone on. Perfect studying habits and work some more on confidence in order to make the next examination experience even better than the last one.

Learn to avoid places where openings occurred for laziness, procrastination and day dreaming.

Use the time between this exam and the next one to better learn to relax, even learning to relax on cue, so that any anxiety can be controlled during the next exam. Learn how to relax the body. Slouch in your chair if that helps. Tighten and then relax all of the different muscle groups, one group at a time, beginning with the feet and then working all the way up to the neck and face. This will ultimately relax the muscles more than they were to begin with. Learn how to breathe deeply and comfortably, and focus on this breathing going in and out as a relaxing thought. With every exhale, repeat the word "relax."

As common as test anxiety is, it is very possible to overcome it. Make yourself one of the test-takers who overcome this frustrating hindrance.

Additional Bonus Material

Due to our efforts to try to keep this book to a manageable length, we've created a link that will give you access to all of your additional bonus material.

Please visit http://www.mometrix.com/bonus948/certhyperbaric to access the information.